# FEEDING

# MY MOTHER

Comfort and Laughter in the Kitchen
as My Mom Lives with Memory Loss

## JANN ARDEN

*Random House Canada*

www.penguinrandomhouse.ca

Random House Canada and colophon are registered trademarks.

Library and Archives Canada Cataloguing in Publication

Arden, Jann, author
Feeding my mother : comfort and laughter in the kitchen as my
mom lives with memory loss / Jann Arden.

Issued in print and electronic formats.
ISBN 978-0-7352-7392-4
eBook ISBN 978-0-7352-7394-8

1. Arden, Jann—Family. 2. Alzheimer's disease—Patients—Care—Alberta.
3. Alzheimer's disease—Patients—Family relationships—Alberta.
4. Mothers and daughters—Alberta. 5. Musicians—Canada—Biography.
6. Caregivers—Alberta—Biography. 7. Alzheimer's disease—
Patients—Alberta—Biography. I. Title.

RC523.2A73 2017      362.1968'3110092      C2017-902276-8

Book design by Terri Nimmo

Photography by Jann Arden. Portraits of Jann and her mom on pages viii, 4–5, 40, 204, 206 and 216 by Nadine Beauchesne, and on page i by Paul Brandt

Illustrations: (65, 79, 161, 196) Terri Nimmo; all others Shutterstock.com: (case, ii–v, 110, 159, 203, 207, 209) Nataliia Kucherenko, (vii, 1–3, 6–7, 34, 90–91, 139, 143, 173, 193, 203, 204–207, 214) Irtsya, (27) Inspiring, (37) Irina Usmanova, (38) Galyna_P, (46) Samburova Maria, (56) ZUBKOVA IULIIA, (87) Elena Medvedeva, (99) runLenarun, (147) Marina Grau, (175, 194) Calesh, (184–185) ru.co.la, (210) lozas, (paper texture) Paladin12, Case background: goldnetz

Printed and bound in Canada

2  4  6  8  9  7  5  3  1

Penguin
Random House
RANDOM HOUSE CANADA

This book is dedicated with an abundance of love and gratitude to
my mom and dad, Joan and Derrel Richards.
Never judgmental.
Always understanding and supportive.
Forever facing forward.

Another year, another page.

A million moments melt away.

The ticking-tocking hands of time,

what's found and lost, remains sublime.

The details that we hold so fast,

are nothing more than memories past.

For love is all that lingers true,

the bond that ties my heart to you.

JANN ARDEN, DECEMBER 29, 2013

*I remember the first day it happened.*

I remember the first time she forgot something big. It wasn't the kind of lapse we all have from time to time— forgetting where we put our keys or our cell phones, or where we parked the car. This was a *big* sudden void. Right after it happened, that morning eight years ago now, I felt a discomfort insert itself at the back of my throat that hasn't really eased up since. It's hard for me to remember what my life used to feel like. It's hard for me to remember my old mom.

We had been sitting having a visit with my sister-in-law, Lori, talking about life things: the weather, the grandkids, jobs, the progress of our summer garden. Everything seemed perfectly normal. My sister-in-law at some point brought up the subject of her old cat. "I didn't want to tell you, Joan," she said to my mom, "but we had to have her put down a few days ago. God, whatever you guys do, don't tell Duray about it as he'll be devastated."

My brother Duray was in jail, as he had been for the last twenty-five years, for first-degree murder—a murder he has always denied committing. He isn't really up to speed on what is going on around our lives out here in the free world, and he's very sensitive to anything the least bit upsetting. I'm sure it's because he feels so helpless. I think that's why Lori wanted to spare him the news about their cat.

"I would *never* say a word," Mom said. Lori went on about how sick the cat had been and that she hadn't found the right moment to tell Duray she was gone. We talked about it in detail for at least fifteen minutes. Mom seemed to be carefully listening to the story, consoling and responding in all the right places. Lori repeated again as she walked out the door, "Please don't say anything, okay, you guys?"

Mom said, "We won't, Lori. Mom's the word." And we all had a bit of a laugh.

Lori waved goodbye, hopped into her little blue compact and pulled out of the driveway.

Before the car had even disappeared down the road, Mom's phone rang, and it was Duray. The first thing that came out of her mouth, was, "You wouldn't believe it, but your cat *died*!" I stood there in her kitchen in disbelief.

"MOM!" I waved my arms in the air trying to get her attention.

"What?" she asked with her hand over the receiver. "I'm *on* the phone!"

"Jesus, you weren't supposed to tell him that!"

"Tell him what?" She looked at me blankly. She really didn't know what she wasn't supposed to tell him.

"About the cat dying! What are you thinking?"


That was the day. From one single second to the next, my life, my mom's life, my dad's life, my brothers' lives, the lives of all of our friends and family, were altered profoundly. My mom had started the journey down the lonely, confusing road called Alzheimer's disease.

I would spend the next two years in denial. I made excuses for both my parents over and over again as the memory thieves slowly stole things from right beneath our noses. I chalked the frequent lapses up to garden-variety old age and tried to leave it at that. My dad had had a stroke several years earlier, so we already knew he had severe memory and mobility issues, but my mom was the normal one. She was the glue that held everything together. She dedicated her days to looking after my dad, coordinating his appointments and doling out his medications. She looked after their house and their yard and their meals and all the driving. I desperately *needed* her to be okay and I was also too scared to think about what was happening.

I must have hoped if I ignored it enough, and wished it away often enough, my mom would start remembering again. But that's not the way Alzheimer's works. I have come to think of it as a cruel and haphazard sculptor. It chisels away at a person, one tiny piece at a time, exposing a mind to every form of loss and sadness. Uncovering every nerve and every bone and every vein. It doesn't stop until it cuts away the last breath. We lived through a small stretch in which my mom knew she was forgetting things. It seemed only a matter of hours to me, but it was actually a short few months where she was aware of things going missing and time being lost and tasks being left undone. She admitted to me once or twice that she knew she was forgetting things. I will never forget her saying to me, "I know I can't remember the way I used to, Jann. It could always be worse, you know. I hope you never let me become a filthy old lady." Those words are stuck inside my heart like wet leaves in a gutter.

I have spent the last few years in various stages of grief and fear and frustration and anger. I'm not sure half the time if I am doing things right with my mom, or screwing things up, but I do know that none of that matters. What matters are the moments spent with the people you love. What matters is setting judgement and resentment aside so that tolerance and patience and kindness can move into your soul and live there in their forever home. Life is never dull. That's what Mom always says. "Life may be hard, but it's not dull . . ."

Mom's journey, and my journey with her, is far from over and for that I am grateful. In these last eight years I have learned more about compassion and empathy and forgiveness than I ever thought possible. I've learned that something good can come from something bad: facing adversity can make you a much better version of yourself. I've learned that having a sense of humour is crucial in order to survive these trying days. I've also learned that feeding my mother, making her a great home-cooked meal, provides both of us with grace and solace and peace, that food is so important for our wellness and contentment. You can soothe pretty much any heartache with a loaf of bread and a hot bowl of soup!

Mom's journey, and my journey with her, is far from over and for that I am grateful.

And I've learned that writing it all down can save me, which is what I started doing when everything around me began to feel unsteady. Seeing what was happening in front of me on the page made it much less daunting. And sharing my thoughts and feelings on social media made all the difference. I guess I wanted to reach out and tell somebody, anybody, about what was happening to my family. I didn't want to feel alone in a room with Alzheimer's. I wanted to throw open every door and window and let the light in. I wanted to unload some of the burden of carrying my parents' secrets. I wanted to rid myself of this weird shame I was feeling because *they* were forgetting themselves. I started feeling like I was being forgotten too, lost in this pile of nothingness. It all seemed like such a mess, and some days it still does. I was talking with a friend about how I was feeling a few months ago, and she described how she felt orphaned when she lost her parents even though she was a grown-up. I think that's exactly how I feel, even though Mom is still here physically. I feel like an orphan.

It turned out that sending out an account of my daily adventures with my folks was life-changing. People started writing back, sharing their doubts and fears and frustrations with me. It changed everything in such a positive, wonderful way. I am so grateful to all of them—to all of you. It takes bravery to share your troubles. It takes grit and guts and gumption. Thank you for easing my troubles, for putting your wisdom and pain out there for everyone to benefit from. I can't tell you how many hours I've spent propped up in my bed reading through the hundreds and hundreds of comments you've left on my Facebook pages. I've laughed out loud and cried quietly and I have to say, I feel much less alone for having reached out. Losing someone an inch at a time is extremely hard.

This book is a glimpse into my journey with memory loss but it's also a journey that thousands and thousands of us are on with our mothers and fathers and sisters and brothers and husbands and wives and uncles and aunts and grandmothers and grandfathers and even children.

Alzheimer's and dementia have always been there, but perhaps families in earlier generations absorbed their elderly folks into the fold of home more gracefully. Many of us these days don't have the kind of lives or rooted family structures that enable us to cope with parents, or grandparents, who can't manage on their own, and we have to find nursing homes for them. Some of these places are great, some not so good, some downright depressing and dehumanizing. It's an agonizing decision and one that can be hard to live with. So far I've been lucky enough to have the means to keep Mom at home with me, and ways to meet the challenges that entails. The stories and the recipes in this book are what I have to share about how we're managing—about the road my mom and all the people who love her are travelling. It was written with humility, and sadness, and fear, and panic, and joy.

What I've learned is that no matter what comes you've got to wrap yourself in all the goodness you can muster. That's what my mom does every single day.

Last week as we were driving into town to buy a few groceries, she told me that she was eighty per cent happy. That made me laugh really hard. "Eighty per cent, Mom? Well, that's way better than me!"

She told me that I would have to work on that . . .

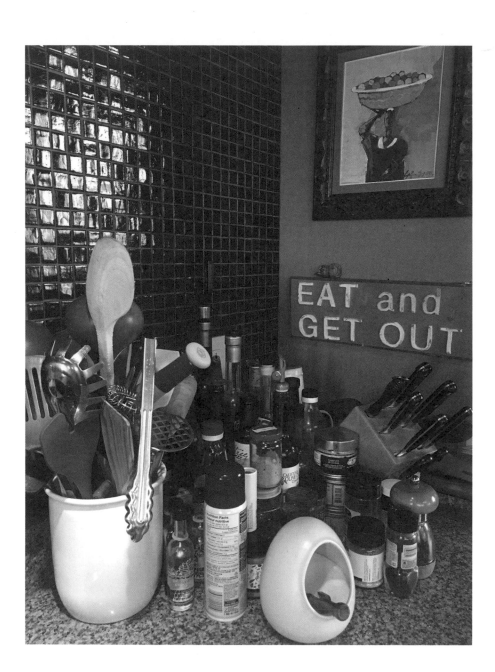

# June 14, 2014

It's been an interesting, daunting, scary, anxiety-ridden week.

Last Wednesday I ended up calling an ambulance to come and

gather up my very delusional, incontinent, falling-all-over-the-

place father. My mom and I had tried to "work through"

whatever issues he was having for about forty-eight hours when

I finally realized that it was something more than him just not

feeling good. He couldn't answer my questions, and when he did

try to answer, his responses were so abstract and zany we

couldn't help but smile (through our fear).

It's difficult watching your parents getting older, and frailer, and increasingly more forgetful. I have watched some of my friends go through similar things with their folks over the past few years, and it's been agonizing to see them with such heavy hearts, so uncertain about what to do next. It's like one moment you are asking for permission to go to a high school dance and the next you're driving into town on a Depends run for your father.

It turns out my dad had some sort of "mystery infection" that triggered the apparent delirium. It's been squashed with antibiotics, but the doctor told us it can take months for an elderly person's mind to clear after such an infection. He has also been diagnosed with dementia, which we more or less knew, as it has come up before in some of his testing. He also has type 2 diabetes and some kidney issues and really crappy circulation in his legs, which makes it hard for him to walk. Other than that, he is super-healthy.

What do we do next?

Well, we want to bring him home. We are just trying to sort out what his needs are going to be once he gets here. So far, I think Mom and I will need:

- a Sherpa to get him up the stairs to his bedroom
- a comedian
- an award-winning food network chef
- a full-time housekeeper
- a butler
- a chauffeur
- a pharmacist
- a team of nurses
- a large oxygen tank
- one of those electric hospital beds
- a soft-serve ice-cream machine
- a gardener
- and a drug dealer for my mother and myself.

Apparently the government will provide us with three hours a week of in-home help of some sort for free. What a load off our shoulders.

Seriously, though, you have to enter this stage of life with a sense of humour. Not only for your aging parents' sakes, but for yourself. Laughter is an amazing love potion and medicine—an incredible healer—and sometimes it's the help you need at the end of a long, hard, delirium-filled day.

## June 15, 2014

My dad called Mom this morning from the hospital and asked her how *she* was. I thought that was adorable. I just need to secure the Sherpa and ice-cream machine and we can bring him home.

## June 17, 2014

Well, my dad gets to come home today. Apparently he is already dressed and sitting on the edge of his bed, ready for us to pick him up.

Every time I went to visit him, he was lying in his bed with his brown leather shoes on. He told me that he was keeping them on his feet because things go missing around there. It made me laugh.

Life is funny. The subject of death can be, too. One day my mom told me that if Dad were to die in the yard, she and I would have to somehow get him into the wheelbarrow and push him up to the house so that the ambulance guys wouldn't have to do it. I am not kidding. Either that, she said, or we'd throw a tarp over him so the dogs wouldn't "get at him." Every time I look at the wheelbarrow now, I smile, thinking of my mom's way of solving problems.

She's never been sentimental. She looks at life with such economy and practicality. She lives in the day and doesn't get too far ahead of herself. When I was nine or ten, she told us at the supper table one night that we would all die one day and that we needed to try and have a happy life. That always stuck with me. To never talk about death is just plain silly. It's like not talking about one of the most important things in our existence.

I hope my dad has a happy summer. I hope he can sit in his lawn chair and yell at me about how I am using the weed eater wrong, or pruning the trees wrong, or hoeing the garden wrong. For some reason, I am looking forward to the old grouch hollering orders at me like I'm some waitress.

## June 25, 2014

My dad has been home just over a week. He is so changed. His facial expressions, even his gestures, are somehow unfamiliar to me—the way his mouth turns down at one corner, the way he looks past you over your shoulder, the way he holds his fork and knife like he is not sure what they're for. The grouchy, strict man who raised three kids, and poured concrete pads his whole life, has left the building. This man is quiet and still, perhaps wondering what his future holds. I catch him standing at the kitchen window looking down the road. His thumbs are shoved through his belt loops, and his jaw moves side to side.

You would think that my mother would be torn apart over losing (more or less) her partner of fifty-six years, but she's steady and calm and goes about her chores around the house without any visible sadness. She'll tell me, "Jann, that's just the way it goes. That's life. What can you do?" She never spends any time feeling sorry for herself—she has bird feeders to fill and squirrels to entertain, after all. She's tied strips of cloth—bits of cut-up tube socks and T-shirts and old aprons—to a dozen tree branches out in the yard. "The squirrels make their beds with them," she answered when I asked what in the hell they were for.

"That's weird, Mom."

"They love them. I put new ones out every few days because they all disappear."

She gets up in the morning and feeds the dogs and putters around. Makes herself and Dad a protein shake with anything that happens to be sitting on the kitchen counter, throwing bananas or nuts or apples into the blender with a scoop of "powder" as she calls it.

She vacuums every single day without fail and does at least one load of laundry. She never says, "I don't know what I'll do without your dad." She always tells me that she'll be fine, though she says she does worry sometimes. But that's what people do. They worry and let their brains run around like chickens in a slaughterhouse. That's what I do, too much of the time.

We are going to try and keep Dad at home. We'll make a few modifications in the bathrooms and we'll bubble-wrap everything. (Kidding.) That has always been the plan.

Mom and I think that Dad will outlive us. He always lands on his feet somehow, the guy who drank and smoked his whole life like some kind of movie star. He still has good days when he makes sense and bad days when we feel like we're playing charades as we try to figure out what he's trying to tell us.

Yesterday he called me and said, "I just wanted to touch base about your financial situation and whatnot." After many failed guesses, I finally figured out he was calling to find out what time I was making him dinner.

*mom and dad*

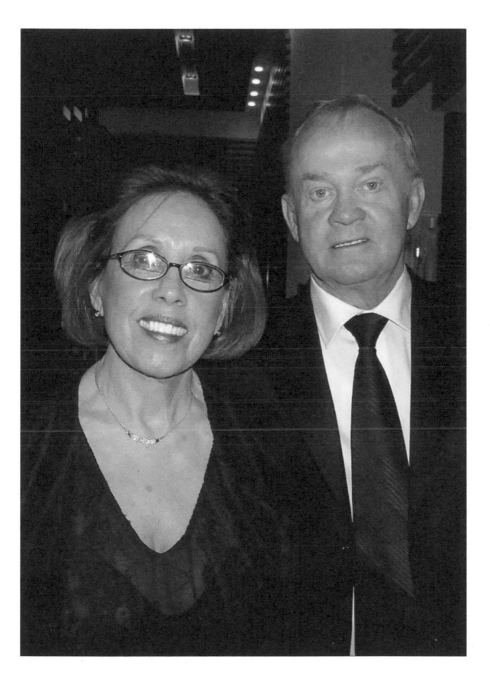

*together for fifty-eight years*

*July 1, 2014*

I have been in Nashville the past few days, getting some writing done and having a little bit of a break from my folks. Though I worry constantly, and I have been calling them three times a day to make sure they are all right.

I keep thinking that I shouldn't have come down here, but Dad seemed to be pretty good. I'll be home on Saturday around suppertime and am hoping that they can keep themselves fed and alive until then.

Of course, as soon as I landed in Nashville, I was getting messages from friends that a tornado had touched down about an hour outside of Calgary. I phoned home to check in, and Mom told me the weather had been so horrible the big dogs ripped the moulding off the door leading from the garage into the house, because they thought the end of the world was upon them. She let them come and lie down on the kitchen floor and took my little Midi upstairs to their walk-in closet.

"Why did you go upstairs, Mom. I thought when a tornado is coming you're supposed to go into the basement?"

"I just thought Midi would like it in there."

"I thought you were finally out of the closet, Mom."

That made her laugh. "Well, I guess not. . ."

Mom has also been giving me daily updates on Midi's bowel movements, which she delivers in a flat, newscaster's voice that makes me laugh every time. "She had a big poo, so that was good." Or, "Dad took her around the yard to poo, but he doesn't know if she did or not, I guess we'll find out."

Mom always says, "There is no news around here," and then proceeds to tell me a long list of things that seem to be of great importance to her.

She and Dad have had the TV stuck on Fox News since I left. "The remote quit working," she told me, which means that my dad probably pressed the wrong button and then kept pressing buttons. I don't even know how to start telling them how to fix it. It's one of those universal remotes that are supposed to be able to tell you what to do if something goes wrong, which is why I got it in the first place.

I don't know what I would do without my friend Donna, who checks on them all the time. Last night she made them chicken and my mom told me it was better than "the stuff I made."

As I hung up the phone from this call, I could hear my dad in the background saying that the goddamn TV was still stuck. My mom began to answer him as she put the phone back in its cradle, and we were cut off. I could picture them in their recliners, staring at that remote control like it was some kind of evil puzzle set by the devil himself.

It's hard being away from home. Not just home I guess, but my family and my friends and my stuff and sometimes my dog(s) and my cat.

I have been travelling for over thirty years for my job and it never gets easier. I have to make sure that I keep up some routines even when I am not waking up in my own house. I have to be mindful of how I am feeling and what I am thinking because it's too easy, when you're away from home, to fall into a slump—not quite

depression, but it could turn into that if I am not mindful of how I am and who I am. I don't want to sound like I sleep in a pyramid wearing healing crystals around my ankles, I only want to stress how important it is to keep a watch on how fast you're running around.

I make sure to take time in the morning to simply lie there for an extra few minutes to prepare myself for my day. I don't turn on the TV or pick up my phone. I just take a minute to say to myself that I am going to be okay and that my day is going to be a good one. It may seem like a small thing, but intention is huge. Intentions are what I am made up of. I intend to do good things and that is something that keeps me balanced and serene.

I always make sure to eat something when I first get up, whether that's an apple stolen from the hotel lobby, an energy bar, a package of cookies from the airplane the day before, a muffin or a bag of peanuts that's been in my purse for a week. You cannot function without food in the morning.

Another thing I do is sit peacefully for a few minutes to try to sort out everything that's going through my brain. I stop to ask myself how I feel. It may seem silly, but how often do you ask yourself that question? *How am I?* A simple thing, but it keeps me sane.

Travelling is not for the frail or weary.

# July 6, 2014

My cat, Sweetpea, is completely blind. I think her hearing is starting to go too. She is nineteen years old, still has pretty great-looking fur, still cleans herself, still spirited even with all her obvious little glitches.

She is, however, peeing and pooping all over the house. I've been putting off the inevitable for two months, torn between having her stay and graciously "letting her go." She loves sitting in the sun. She still loves to roll in catnip—I put out so much for her she always looks like she's covered in oregano—and have her chin scratched. Even though I want her to have one last great summer, the "waste" issue is wearing me down. Though maybe it's partly my fault: I have been giving her a lot of treats and feeding her as much cat food as she wants, whenever she wants.

I know some people would say, "Hey, don't feel guilty, it's just what has to be done." But I do feel guilty. Thinking about having the vet come here to deliver that ever-so-final little prick that allows her to drift off to forever land keeps me awake at night. I feel like I am facing two really bad choices.

I am watching Sweetpea now. She's circling the kitchen floor and bumping into the chairs like a furry pinball machine. It makes me smile, although it's not that funny, especially not for her. She is trying to find her way back to her couch, which I've covered with old bedsheets because she sheds so much. She is having a harder and harder time figuring out where her bed is. I feel like I am watching her decline inch by inch, unable to make that phone call to my trusted vet, my dear friend Judith.

I wish I could find the simple strength to do the right thing. This really sucks.

## July 13, 2014

Of course I always knew that my parents would get older, that things would change. But I wasn't prepared for how much they would change and how quickly. It's been uplifting and heartbreaking and mind-boggling watching what a fifty-six-year marriage means to two people when things start to fall apart, and how adaptable those two people have to be.

My parents do this kind of dance in the house, weaving in and around each other without really having to think about who will move where or how or when. It is a dance created over time, through practice and repetition. By this point they read each other through a glance, even a shift in breathing.

"I can tell he's asleep by how he's breathing," my mom will say. "I can tell if he's sick by the way his face changes colour. You wouldn't notice, but I do. . . ."

Last night, my dad was staring at my mom's teacup, which was sitting to one side of her dinner plate. I thought to myself, *What the hell is he thinking about?* My mom glanced up at me and said, "He wants a glass of water." He nodded and looked at me as if to say, "What took you so long to figure that out, you silly goose?"

Through all the anger and disappointment that they've faced, they have somehow managed to maintain a precarious balance of peace between them. Even facing the brutal reality of my older brother being in jail for all these years, they stand in a lonesome solidarity that no one else can even begin to understand. They've never turned any of their lives' calamities into resentment or hatred. These days, couples seem to split up at the first sign of any trouble. My mother has said to me on more than one occasion that she doesn't always like my dad, but she always loves him. That has always made so much sense to me. There are days when I don't like him either, but my love for him is constant.

He is grouchy a lot of the time, and ungrateful, and when he doesn't want to answer a question, completely unresponsive. I end up getting mad, but I look at my mother and she is always calm. "I just ignore him," she'll say to me. "Don't let him get to you." And then she grabs a handful of peanuts and heads out to feed the squirrels who wait for her like she is Jesus returning. They get so excited I always worry about them leaping right into her apron. I watch them rub their little hands together like they're praying, and exulting, "We are saved!"

My parents are the last of a dying breed. There is a joke in there somewhere, and I will figure it out eventually. They are an old-school couple who have made their way courageously through life, never feeling sorry for themselves, finding grace in the small things. And always going forward. No matter what.

One of those small reliable things that hasn't changed with my parents is the simple joy of having a good meal together. It's something they look forward to—my dad especially. I started cooking regularly for them after several trips over to their place to help them to "figure out this goddamn can opener." My dad has always had a way with words. I was marching home in a bit of a huff after opening the third can of chunky soup in as many days—wondering why the heck they were eating so many meals from a can—when it dawned on me: heating up a can of soup was something my mom could still manage to do.

I started by cooking dinner for them once or twice a week. Within a month, they were coming arm in arm across the driveway towards my house almost every evening, chattering away like two old birds chirping on a wire. It was all they could do to wait until five-thirty. If Dad had had his way, he would have been on my doorstep by three.

I hadn't really done a lot of cooking in my life. I mean I cooked, but pretty much the same five or six things over and over again. My job has always meant that I eat out—a lot! Now I had to figure out how to prepare nutritious but fun meals that Mom and Dad would enjoy. Thank heaven for the inspiration of cooking shows. Luckily for me, my folks would try anything I put in front of them and they always seemed to like it. The other wrinkle was that I rarely had the time to spend three hours putting together a difficult recipe, so I eventually adapted many of my favourite dishes so that making them was simple and easy. Like this one, for example, my turkey chili.

# TURKEY CHILI

3 tbsp olive oil

1 onion, chopped

1 lb ground turkey or
veggie crumbles

3 tbsp chilli powder

1 tsp cumin

1 tbsp salt

1 19 oz (540 mL) can
diced tomatoes, with
their juice

1 19 oz (540 mL) can
kidney beans, rinsed
and drained

1 19 oz (540 mL) can
black beans, rinsed
and drained

¼ cup ketchup

2 tbsp balsamic vinegar

1 tsp sugar

This recipe can totally be vegetarian—just swap the turkey for veggie crumbles, which you'll find in the produce section of your grocery store. It's great on its own or over rice, pasta or baked potato.

Set a large, deep sided frying pan over medium heat. Add the oil, onions and turkey (or veggie crumbles) and get it all browning. Add the chili powder, cumin and salt and stir well to coat everything.

When your turkey and onions are cooked through, add the tomatoes and beans, ketchup, vinegar and sugar. Simmer for 30 minutes. If you like, serve with a dollop of sour cream or a handful of shredded cheddar. Dad liked both.

# July 18, 2014

When tragedies happen now, they feel both global and incredibly personal. It's like a shard of grief pierces the hearts of people all around the world at the same time and unites us for a moment, crossing all borders, all ethnic lines, all colours and religious beliefs. We are bound together for that moment by an incredible wave of compassion and loss and empathy for people we do not know, but feel a connection with. More than a connection—we ARE those people. Even if it's just for a breath or two, we are those who are lost and we wince with a surreal kind of shock. Who could do this? What makes people so evil?

I walked the dog down the road this morning after a terrible night's sleep. Syria, refugees drowning in the Mediterranean. I listened to the crunch of gravel beneath my feet and squinted into the sun, filled with a dull kind of agony. I actually told Midi, right out loud, that she was lucky she didn't know what was going on in the world.

I couldn't get the pictures out of my head: clouds of thick black smoke billowing up into the bluest of skies, vast fields of grass that had been waiting to be cut, now burning. Such a juxtaposition of everything good and everything bad. Little shoes sitting beside a scattered deck of playing cards, a leather purse, a passport, a suitcase perfectly intact, waiting for its owner to claim it.

As the dog and I walked home with the wind at our backs and the sun streaking through the trees, I thought to myself how good people are. How kind and helpful and hard-working and empathetic. Even though my faith in the human race is challenged at every turn, I still believe that goodness is abundant and that bad people will not be able to turn us into the bitter, hateful souls they seem to want us to be. They want us to be like them, full of dark and dread and doom, to become wicked beings set on causing pain for the sake of pain. I will find the good people and I will surround myself with them. I'll keep trying to be decent and thoughtful and helpful and creative. I'll leave good things behind me when I pass. I promise this to myself.

# July 27, 2014

I went over to my parents' house yesterday because they needed me to open a can of ham. My dad thought he had really lost his marbles but, honestly, I couldn't get that f&*%ing can to open myself. I told him it had nothing to do with him, that this time it *was* the bloody can opener's fault. He was *so* relieved. "Well, let's throw it out," he said.

"We can't throw out a perfectly good can opener!" I said.

"Yes, we can. Your mother and I threw out the coffee pot last week, so we can throw this out too."

"You threw out the coffee pot?"

"It wasn't working."

"You should have called me to come over."

"Your mother doesn't want you to think we're crazy."

"Well, it's too late for that, Dad. . . ."

My mom started laughing her head off.

The simplest things are getting complicated. Just when you think you're at an age when you've pretty much got life figured out, you forget what you're doing. You forget how to make the string longer on the weed-eater. You forget how to set the clock radio. You forget how to pop the gas thingy open on your car so you can fill it up.

It's these things that bother my parents most of all, not the fact that Dad can't walk to the mailbox anymore, or that he doesn't sleep well, or that he can't drive his truck. It's not being able to open a damn can of ham.

After they threw out their perfectly good coffee pot, they headed straight over to Walmart and bought a Keurig coffee brewer. They can't figure that out.

A friend printed out a very large set of instructions and taped them onto the cabinet door, and they STILL can't figure it out.

My dad was a person who could have assembled a helicopter if he put his mind to it. He could do or make anything—build houses and rebuild truck engines and make delicate rocking chairs and tables and birdhouses. So it's hard to watch him struggling with a can opener or making a cup of coffee. It's harder, still, knowing my parents feel ashamed about not being able to figure out those simple things.

"I don't know how you do all that stuff on your phone," my mom said to me one morning. I don't know how myself, to tell you the truth. I just figured out how to change my ringtone a month ago. It had been some kind of minstrel-sounding harp for the previous fifteen months.

Even though they are fighting their way through their own maze most days, they still find humour in everything. Mom was feeding the dogs saltine crackers this morning, right out of the package.

"Are the crackers stale, Mom?" I wondered.

"I doubt it."

"I mean, can't you guys still eat them?"

"I don't know." And then she laughed and got up and walked outside and fed a handful of old cupcake bits and some bacon to the squirrel who had been waiting for her all morning.

## August 6, 2014

I finally found the courage to have Sweetpea put down. I went back and forth so many times trying to come to terms with what I had to do. I guess I hoped that one morning I would wake up and find my old cat curled up in her favourite bed, already gone to heaven. But when the weight started coming off her and her hearing went the way of her sight, I knew it was already past the point where I needed to show her some grace.

My mom helped me bury her on a ridge behind the house, both of us crying as we shovelled dirt over that little cardboard box. I'd wrapped her in a fuzzy towel. Then we said a prayer and stood looking out over the river. There were birds singing particularly loud and sweet, just for Sweetpea, I like to think. The wind was warm and slow, and the trees waved back and forth with a slow and steady solidarity, like pallbearers. I hardly slept last night, riddled with guilt, not because I'd finally asked the vet to come but because I have been away so much over the years. Sweetpea was left alone in the house a lot after her two companions died. It was just Sweetpea, roaming around, keeping the mouse population in line. We always left music on for her, a lovely classical mix. Dad would say, "What if she likes country?" I would look at him and shrug and say, "Dad, no one likes country that much. . . ."

Afterwards, when I called Mom to tell her that Sweetpea was gone, she simply said, "Well, isn't it nice to know that she can see again?"

Yes, it is, I said. It really is.

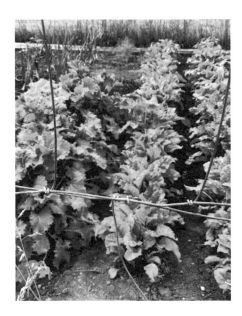

# August 19, 2014

My parents left the hose on all night in the front yard so the trees got a *really* good drink. When I mentioned it to Mom this morning, I thought she was going to cry. I told her it was fine, that the lawn needed a good watering. She said she'd just forgotten it was on. It can happen to anyone—a few weeks ago I was watering a new tree near my driveway and forgot the hose was on for six hours.

I try to not make them feel like the world is ending, but it's hard some days. I feel like my voice is raised and my hands are flying around and my body language is saying, "What the hell are you guys doing over here?" I know that worrying and nagging doesn't do anything but make you sick and tired and lacking in joy. I don't want to be that person. My parents are managing pretty well, all things considered. We'll just muddle through this, one day at a time, or maybe it should be a couple of hours at a time. All I can do is somehow find it in myself to accept all the little changes that are happening. I find it comforting on so many levels just to spend quality time with Mom and Dad. Even *I* am surprised by how wonderful it is to simply sit down and share a meal at the same table. I mean, over the past decade we only really had meals together at Christmas and Easter. This is all new for me; for an hour or two, time seems to stop and I feel like it's 1985.

Last night we had a bit of buffet. Mom loves her veggies and she was happy about the salads I made. I also decided to serve up my special tuna dish, which is so great when it's hot.

# WATERMELON, RED ONION, FETA AND MINT SALAD WITH LIME AND HONEY DRESSING

4 cups roughly chopped watermelon, well chilled

1 medium red onion, thinly sliced

1 cup crumbled feta cheese

1 cup torn mint leaves

## DRESSING:

juice of 1 lime

2 tbsp honey

2 tbsp white wine vinegar or apple cider vinegar

pinch salt

Get a large bowl and throw in your chopped watermelon, sliced onion, mint and feta. Toss gently, so as to not mush up your watermelon. Set aside.

I use a jar with a lid to shake up my dressing, but you could also mix it in a small bowl. Juice your lime, add your honey and vinegar and pinch of salt, and mix or shake well. Pour over your salad and be sure to coat everything as evenly as possible—you don't need very much dressing. Even though it doesn't look like a lot, it's plenty!

Serve it straight away—this salad can't sit for very long, as it starts to wilt immediately.

# FENNEL, GREEN ONION AND RADISH SLAW WITH CREAMY, SPICY PEANUT DRESSING

3 large fennel bulbs, trimmed and thinly sliced (save a few fronds for garnish)

10–15 radishes, thinly sliced

2–3 green onions, sliced into small pieces

¼ cup chopped peanuts (I like salted ones)

### DRESSING:

¼ cup peanut butter

¼ cup rice vinegar, or to taste

1 tbsp fish sauce

½ tsp salt

½ tsp cayenne

½ tsp sesame oil

I use the common round red radishes, but you can use any type of radish you have on hand. I have used a mandolin and I've used my food processor and I've done it by hand with a sharp knife—slice the fennel and radishes any way you choose, just don't chop your darn fingers off.

To make the dressing, put everything in a small bowl and mix very well. It takes some elbow grease for sure. It's very thick to start off with, but loosens up as you get going. Set aside, then give it another quick mix before you pour the whole works over your salad.

Take your sliced fennel, radish and green onion, and put them in a large bowl. Mix them up with your fingers. Toss with the dressing.

Chop up some of the fennel fronds you've saved and sprinkle over each serving of salad. Add some crushed peanuts on each dish as well—as little or as much as you like.

# AHI TUNA WITH
# ROASTED GARLIC CHIPS AND
# HOISIN HOT SAUCE

¼ cup hoisin sauce

2 tbsp hot sauce

1 tsp sesame oil

2 tbsp coconut oil

8 garlic cloves, sliced as thinly as possible without cutting your fingers off

1 8 oz filet sushi grade tuna (I'm warning you, it's expensive, but sometimes just what you need)

salt and pepper

In a small bowl stir together your hoisin, hot sauce and sesame oil. Set aside.

You'll want to put a frying pan big enough to fit the entire piece of tuna over high heat. Add the coconut oil and your thinly sliced garlic. WATCH IT LIKE A HAWK. It will go brown almost instantly. As soon as it's golden, get it out of the pan and onto a paper towel.

Season your tuna steak with salt and pepper and put it into the pan. This, too, will cook very quickly. You don't really want to do anything but SEAR the steak—no more than 90 seconds a side. Remove from heat and let it rest for a few minutes. Now slice the tuna into bite-sized pieces. Spoon on some of your hoisin mixture and top with a few garlic chips. Serve at room temp with some stir-fried veggies in winter, or salads like the two on the previous pages.

## August 21, 2014

I'm about to go on tour, and I keep running through
the upcoming show in my head. I picture myself out
there on stage as every possible thing goes wrong. My
clothes fall off, I forget lyrics, I trip into the orchestra
pit, my hair catches on fire, the band goes on stage
completely plastered. I worry this way every single
time I head out on the road.

The worst hours are between 3 and 5 a.m. After my
mind wanders through every possible performing
disaster, it moves merrily on to the fragile yet
humorous state my folks find themselves in these days.
Then I enter the weird zone where I count heartbeats,
think about my future, my past—why I never had
children, how I am going to die—then count more
heartbeats and obsess about a developer who is
planning a massive housing project on my beloved
road. I run through the entire spectrum of horrors that
my brain can conjure up.

At this point in the game last night, I managed to talk
myself into getting up and working out, which I SO
did NOT want to do. Once I got going, though, I felt
better. There is something about sweating out one's
troubles that makes it worth it to climb ten thousand
imaginary stairs.

After I had showered and fed the dog, I walked over to
Mom and Dad's.

Mom said, as I came in, "You look tired. You're kind of a funny colour."

That is always nice to hear.

She knew by the look on my face that she should follow with something a bit more upbeat. "Well, Dad and I thought we could take you to the buffet tonight at the Casino."

I wanted to go back to the funny-colour comment. "What do you mean, funny?"

"Have you been suntanning?"

"No," I said, "I have not been suntanning." Under my breath, I muttered that I could probably manage a buffet even though I was a weird colour.

But Mom overheard me and had a helpful suggestion. "You could wear a hat and some glasses so that nobody would notice."

Thank you. Thank you very much. Wearing a hat and sunglasses to an Asian buffet at seven o'clock at night never attracts attention.

# September 13, 2014

I have been meaning to write for two weeks, but life on the road tends to capture your entire being and hold it hostage. I find it hard to sleep on the bus, even with Midi snoring away at the foot of my bunk. I am envious of her ability to travel so effortlessly. Maybe if I was her size and could fit in a purse.

Even when I was younger, I could not for the life of me fall asleep on a tour bus. Imagine being in a long dark box that is really noisy and pitches from side to side as it barrels along at ninety kilometres an hour.

People always think it's so glamorous on the damn bus, but the bus is like camping without ever being able to stop.

On the day I left, my mom had to call 911 and have Dad taken to the hospital (where else, pray tell, do you take a person in an ambulance?). It was a giant shit show just as I was about to get on the plane, and I was completely torn. But my little brother, Patrick, and his wonderful girlfriend, Jodi, and my dear friend Theresa completely stepped up and looked after everything for me. I am so blessed to have people in my life who are dependable and loyal and trustworthy. I don't think I could have carried on with the tour if it weren't for them. You really do find out who your friends are when tragedy strikes and the ball drops and the bull wanders into the china shop!

Anyway Dad came home again a few days later, thank heavens.

Life really is moment to moment. I know I can't live too far in the future, because it just makes me anxious. I tell myself to deal with where I am and what's happening in the moment. I called Mom a little while ago and she said Dad was quiet today. Perhaps he is thinking about life trickling by. . . .

I am literally going to go and get on the stage right now. That's living in the moment.

# October 2, 2014

I made it home last night and it is so very quiet around here. I had gotten used to being around twenty-four people at all times, eating with them, sleeping with them (you know what I mean—on the bus), laughing with them, crying with them, creating with them.

My band was, as always, brilliant. Keith, Pat, Allison, Graham, Darcy, Kristyn, Mike—what a dream team. My crew was amazing too, leaving no detail to chance. I am blown away by what they do, and how well they do it. Every night I stood on that stage was pure magic. If you've ever doubted that the universe has a God, music is a reminder that there is one. I don't know what that means, or what it is, or who it is, but I am amazed and humbled by whatever or whoever has put this all together.

 I got up this morning and went out to the garden to dig up my potatoes, onions and carrots. I had to leave them in the ground when I left for Victoria to start the tour, but they all survived. I am making Mom and Dad roasted root veggies and turkey meatloaf for dinner tonight. They both look great and are in good spirits. When I walked into their house last night, they both stood up to greet me (which made me want to cry), then Dad said, "We're still alive!" Then Mom said, "Well, just barely . . ." And then we all laughed. Alive indeed.

I made them turkey meatloaf for dinner, and Dad carried home the leftovers.

*sometimes I need my treehouse refuge*

# TURKEY MEATLOAF
# WITH ZUCCHINI AND CARROTS

1 lb ground turkey

1 egg

1 small zucchini, grated

1 small white onion, diced

1 carrot, grated

1 garlic clove, minced

¼ cup ketchup

2 tbsp sriracha

2 tbsp olive oil

2 tbsp soy sauce

1 tbsp Worcestershire sauce

salt and pepper

½ cup bread crumbs (you can use ground flax instead, but it's got a very distinct taste so beware. . . . I love it, but some people hate it.)

The great thing about this recipe is that you can put everything into one large bowl . . . and it's got tons of veggies that people won't even know they're eating.

Preheat the oven to 375°F. Get an 8x4-inch loaf pan ready . . . greased and floured, or use parchment paper like I always do.

Roll up your sleeves. In a large bowl, get mixing with your hands and, in my case, wrists. Incorporate everything together and then transfer your "meat ball" into your loaf pan and stick it into the oven for 50 minutes.

Some people make a glaze out of equal parts ketchup and corn syrup, but honestly I would rather just eat it on its own. Mom likes having this recipe with a can of beans and some tomato slices. It's never too fancy around our house.

# October 8, 2014

There are days when I feel like I am the worst person in the world. I sit in a chair and feel like everything I do and everything I say is mean-spirited and selfish. When it comes to the care of my mom and dad, this is the weight that slithers my way on occasion. Both of them are now all over the place when it comes to their memories and I find myself getting more and more impatient—more snippy, more grumpy, more frustrated.

Mom said to me the other day, "You always seem mad at me, Jann. . . ." I died a little inside after she let that sentence fall out of her mouth. I told her I wasn't mad, that I was just caught off guard with this new version of them.

"This is new to me too," she said. "And I can't do a darn thing about it. I am practically drinking that coconut oil you bought us."

That really made me laugh. I told her that I hoped she was kidding.

But I loathe watching them misplace every single thing: keys and purses and credit cards and hats and coats and money and electric bills and coffee mugs and glasses and the TV remote. There are elves in the house, "movers," my mom calls them, who take things and put them just out of reach, just out of plain sight.

"The movers move things," she said a little while ago. "Either that or your dad and I are going crazy. At least we're doing it together."

They are indeed doing it together. They *never* get mad at each other. My dad will answer the same question from my mom a hundred times and not even flinch. I lash out like a whip after about the fourth time Mom asks me something and then feel completely ashamed. I called her the other day and told her how sorry I was and she said, "About what?" It gave me a lump in my throat the size of a toaster.

"About me being so short with you."

"Well, you're doing the best you can. You always do and we appreciate everything you do. . . ."

When she lets me off the hook that way, I can feel my heart pump the blood to the end of my fingers. I can feel it fill my cheeks and pulse in my running shoes that are tied too tight again.

My mom is so kind. It baffles me how my dad's drinking and carrying on back in the day didn't make her coarse and bitter and unmerciful. No matter how much he yelled, or how drunk he got, or how often he stormed around like a four-year-old, my mom just kept right on being herself: empathetic, good-natured, generous, funny and thoughtful. And here I am, turning into some kind of memory referee, blowing my whistle and crying foul every time either of them repeat themselves or get mixed up.

After much reflection, I have realized how scared I am. I am scared of them forgetting themselves and taking me with them into oblivion. I am scared of how their lives seem to be stolen day by day, their shared past thrown into a blender. I am just scared.

The funny part of all of it is that they aren't the least bit concerned. They don't seem scared at all. They are happy. They are light-hearted and positive and faithful and easygoing. I am the only one freaking out.

I need to tear a page out of their book and just calm the hell down. So what if they put the remote in the fridge? So what if the car keys are in with the dog food?

As Mom said, "We find things eventually, Jann. It's not the end of the world."

After much
reflection,
I have
realized how
scared I am.

# October 11, 2014

I spent the afternoon yesterday in the yard with my parents. There was something about the autumn leaves falling from the poplars through the sun, like thin gold coins, that eased my heart. Everything seemed so familiar and easy. It made me think of my childhood, when life was a hell of a lot more straightforward.

My mother did warn my brothers and me about what was coming. She told us one similar fall afternoon, many years ago, that we'd have to fend for ourselves someday, buy our own toothpaste and toilet paper, that she and Dad wouldn't always be there to do everything. We were standing out in the yard leaning on our shovels and rakes. Mom and Dad had us all working in the garden and we hated every second of it.

*Yeah, right*, I thought to myself. *Like that will ever happen.*

None of us thought it would ever be any different that it was that crisp day. We would be looked after forever. That memory feels like a shard of beautiful glass piercing me.

Yesterday the air was cool enough for us to need our old sweaters and ball caps. Mom was wearing one from 1994 that says "Insensitive."

"You STILL have that crazy old hat," I said to her.

"What hat?"

"The one that's on your head."

"What's the matter with it?"

"It says 'Insensitive.'"

"And . . . ?"

"It's just funny that you still have it."

"I have everything I ever had," she said, matter-of-factly.

And she may be right, because my parents' house is starting to look cluttered. Not terribly, yet, but you can see the wave beginning to gather speed.

The clutter started in the closet upstairs and now it's creeping down the hall into the laundry room. Piles of magazines and all kinds of rags. Hundreds of bits of paper with random things written on them.

I recently picked up a pile that was sitting on the dryer and shuffled my way through it. One note read, "owe jann 19 dollars." It was dated last July. I stood there wondering what she owed me nineteen dollars for.

Mom started laughing when I asked her why she was saving all this crap. She said, "I just need it and I don't know why. So there. You can burn it all when I die."

"Maybe I will burn it, or maybe I'll sell it all on eBay."

"You should just have a big yard sale. You could wait a few months at least after I'm dead. . . ."

"I'll wait at least three months."

"Good."

"Fine."

Then we both laughed and Dad told us we needed to get back to work. And then he laughed too.

We spent the rest of the day gathering up the potatoes and the carrots and onions, rubbing off most of the dirt and putting them down in the root cellar. Dad built it himself years ago and it's still rock solid. I marvel at what that guy could do. Literally anything.

It felt good to get it all done before the winter sets in.

It felt good to see Mom and Dad out in the yard.

I tried to stop time with my head and make the moment freeze. The two of them chatting back and forth, taking exactly one second at a time.

That night we ate roasted root vegetables from the garden, and this:

# CHICKEN PARM
# (THAT ANYBODY CAN MAKE)

4 boneless, skinless chicken breasts

1 cup panko or dry bread crumbs (I have even used crumbled corn flakes in a pinch)

1 tsp cayenne

1 tsp salt

1 tsp pepper

1 tsp oregano

1 tsp garlic salt

2 eggs

1 cup shredded mozzarella

½ cup grated Parmesan

1 jar of your favourite spaghetti sauce (honestly, who has the time?)

I also added a side of sautéed mushrooms . . . I love that combo.

Preheat your oven to 425°F.

Put each individual breast into a resealable bag. I use a rolling pin to pound the breasts down into a flatter version of themselves. Put the panko in a large bowl with ALL the spices. Mix well.

Beat the eggs in a separate bowl big enough to dip the chicken breasts into without making a complete mess. Dip each piece, shake off the excess egg, then dip into the panko and cover them completely. Set them on a sheet pan covered with some parchment paper . . . you HAVE to have some parchment, otherwise it's a nightmare to clean!

Put the chicken in the oven for 18 to 20 minutes. Remove the chicken at that point and cover each breast with a dollop of tomato sauce (from a jar of your favourite spaghetti sauce) and a big handful of the mozzarella and Parmesan. Put them back into the oven for 5 to 6 minutes. (Then I like to put them under the broiler for 60 seconds at the end to get the cheese kind of burned. Well, not quite . . . you don't have to do this last step, unless you love that almost crispy and golden cheese as much as I do.)

# November 1, 2014

As soon as I walked through the door at my parents' place, I spotted Mom's new wallet open on the side table with nothing in it . . . well, nothing but her Indigo/Chapters reward card. For the last three weeks I have been shuttling Mom all over town trying to get all her ID replaced after she lost her purse and had no idea where or why or how ("I think your dad left it at the coffee place . . ."). I was hoping to find it stuffed in a birdhouse or in the dryer or in the garage or in the dog food bag, where a lot of lost items turn up, but no such luck. Credit cards, health care card, driver's licence, pacemaker cards, birth certificate—everything was gone.

It is no simple task getting everything back, let me tell you. Thank God my dad had their passports tucked away in his sock drawer, because that became my key to being able to replace everything without having to resort to crying my head off at the registrar's office.

So, long story longer, before I left on a business trip last week, I had it all dealt with. I felt a huge sense of accomplishment and relief. I told Mom how important it was to put everything back in her wallet after she used it AND to put her wallet back in her purse. Then I saw it sitting there with nothing in it and I could hear my own voice rise into the air like cheap fireworks. "Where the hell are all your cards, Mom?!"

"What cards?"

"All your credit cards! All the stuff we replaced before I left!" My tone was more an angry colour than a sound.

"Why would I take my cards out of there? I don't remember doing that. I don't know where they are, Jann. They are somewhere, though. I bet they are in my purse."

She started rummaging through all the coats and scarves hung on hooks by the back door. I stood over her like a prison guard and said, "Don't you have someplace you put your purse every day?" Being bossy is unbecoming of anyone, and is not my nature at all. I hate the new me.

As she kept searching through the coats, she said, "It was nice not having anybody yell at me this last month. Your dad's half crazy, but he doesn't ever yell."

I was immediately filled with regret and shame. "I was only gone a week."

"Well, it felt like a lot longer."

She finally found her little red purse and started pulling things out if it. Kleenexes and hand lotion, a comb, more tissues, a toothbrush, a mirror, her cell phone (for which they'd been looking for days), a handful of loose change and finally a little stack of cards. "There, see?" she said.

I felt stupid and small. Again. "Why didn't you put them back in your wallet? You're going to give me a heart attack!"

"You're going to give *yourself* a heart attack, Jann."

"I just don't want you to lose all your stuff again."

"Well, I might. That's just how it goes when you're old. And if I do, we can go get them all again. I can go and do it with your dad—we don't mind. But I found them, so there."

I told her I was sorry, and that I didn't mean to raise my voice. Then my dad came in and sat at the kitchen table and asked me what was for lunch, like he hadn't seen or heard anything that had been going on. I picked up Midi, and walked over and handed her to him. He warmed her little feet in his hands.

"Do you want me to make you some lunch?" I asked him.

"Sure," he said, grinning from ear to ear. "Whaddaya got?"

"Whadda*you* got?"

"I'll eat whatever you want to make me."

"How about alligator?"

"Fine."

"Alligator it is."

Then my mom came into the kitchen clutching all her stuff in her hands and looking all over the place for something.

"What are you doing?" I said.

"Looking for my wallet."

I didn't make alligator, but warmed up some of my "stewp," and toasted slices of the cheese and onion herb bread I like to make.

# CHEESE AND ONION
# HERB BREAD

½ cup milk

½ cup water

2 tbsp butter

2 cups all-purpose flour

1 tsp fast-rising yeast

1 tsp sugar

1 tsp salt

1 egg

1 cup grated cheese
(you can do two or
three kinds to make up
the cup if you want)

2 green onions, finely
chopped

A handful of chopped
fresh herbs. Dill and
thyme work really well.

**Super easy. You can throw in any herb you love. Best of all, you don't have to be a baker to make this stuff.**

Set a saucepan over medium heat. Add the milk, water and butter and heat until the butter melts; set aside.

In a giant bowl, combine one cup of the flour with the yeast, sugar and salt. Stir the dry stuff together really well.

Crack the egg into the dry mixture, break it up with a fork and stir it around for a few seconds. Now add all your milk-water-butter mixture. Roll your sleeves up and start kneading everything together IN the bowl, adding the cheese, green onions, the herbs and some more of the flour. You want to make a nice ball—NOT too hard, NOT too much flour. You may not use the entire other cup of flour . . . I usually don't.

You don't have to take it out of the bowl, which is why I like this recipe—it's NOT messy. Keep kneading the dough in the bowl for a few minutes and make a nice ball. Set aside at room temperature for about an hour or so (you can cover the top of the bowl with a tea towel if you like). Preheat your oven to 350°F.

Transfer your dough into a well-greased and floured cake or loaf pan depending on whether you'd like a round or a rectangle loaf, or whatever you've got on hand. I have even done little separate buns in a muffin tin. I usually cut a cross into the top of the dough with a sharp knife, which makes it rise a little better in my opinion.

Bake for 50 minutes, or 22–25 minutes if you're doing the muffin version. Keep an eye on the bread, and remove when slightly browned.

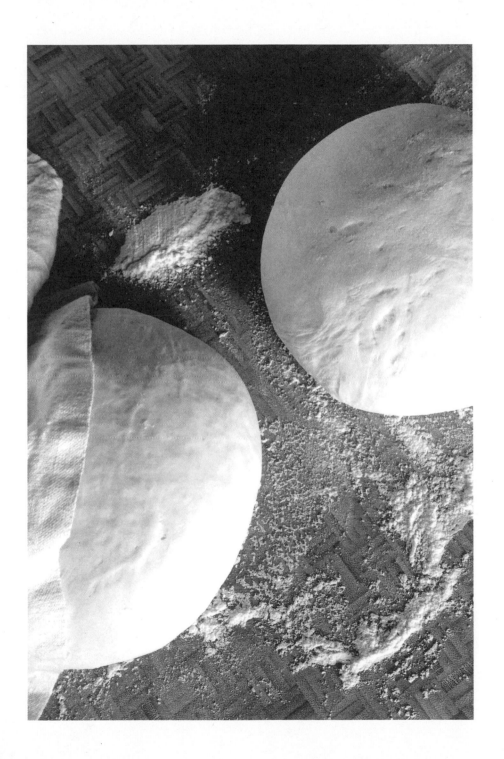

# FOUR-BEAN VEGETABLE "STEWP"

¼ cup coconut oil or
   olive oil

1 medium onion, roughly
   chopped

1 medium red pepper,
   finely chopped

1 carrot, finely chopped

1 cup green beans,
   trimmed

1 garlic clove, crushed

1 tsp mild curry powder

1 tsp cumin

2 tsp salt

1 tsp pepper

1 tbsp apple cider
   vinegar, or to taste

1 19 oz (540 mL) can
   black beans, rinsed
   and drained

1 19 oz (540 mL) can
   kidney beans, rinsed
   and drained

1 19 oz (540 mL) can
   pinto beans, rinsed
   and drained

1 19 oz (540 mL) can
   stewed tomatoes, with
   their juice

2 tbsp ketchup

4 cups (1 L) water

You can use any beans that you want here—just drain and rinse them well. Don't use lentils—it's not the flavour we're going for in this recipe. It's a great stew to freeze—often I'll double it so I have extra.

Set a large, deep sided frying pan over medium heat. Add coconut oil and all your chopped veggies, garlic, spices, salt and pepper, and stir them together well. Splash in your vinegar and sauté for at least 5 minutes, or until your onions are translucent. Add the tomatoes with their juices along with the beans, ketchup and water.

Simmer it all for 45 minutes. (This recipe is also great in a slow cooker—throw everything in and set it on low for 6 hours.) I usually make it in the morning and leave it on low for a few hours.

Serve with a chunk of the herb bread, or any crusty loaf, to sop up all those great flavours.

{ 65 }

## November 8, 2014

I was away again this week, and my parents did well. I left Midi with them and I think they would rather have her sitting in their kitchen than me.

I called them every day to check up on the pill taking and dog walking and the meals they were having and how everybody was sleeping and if I had any mail and what the neighbourhood news was. (Dad gets up at two in the morning every night and goes downstairs to sleep in his chair, which is why I always ask about the sleeping thing.) Every day, Mom would tell me that nothing was new around there and that nobody had died. "We're all alive so that's good!" she'd say, and then laugh this adorable laugh, and a wave of relief would wash over me.

Not dead indeed. My parents don't live in the future ever. I seem to constantly be living in a day that isn't here yet. They always deal with the hour they are living in. They don't get ahead of themselves, they don't worry, they don't lament or dread what may or may not be coming their way. I need to get to that place, and sooner rather than later.

And my mom is so funny, she really is. When I call, she always tells me two things right off the top: whether Midi had a poop, and what they had for dinner. The other night she told me that she and Dad split a ham sandwich and that dad's half was bigger than hers. "He can sure eat . . ." she said and I could hear her roll her eyes. "He ate the last cinnamon bun this morning, too, and didn't even ask me if I wanted a bite!" And then I heard Dad yell at her from across the living room because he always listens to every word she says to me. "I gave you HALF of that bun, Mother!"

"You did? Well, your dad just told me that he gave me half of his cinnamon bun. I guess I forgot." And they both laughed like little kids.

"Yes, you had half of that bun and you had a big piece of my fudge too!"

They often talk back and forth when I call and I just hang on the other end of the line and listen to them chatter.

I said, "Hello, Mom. Do you want to hang up?"

"No."

"Okay, well, you were talking to dad and I just thought you wanted to get going."

"It's the only time he listens to me . . ."

"Why is that?"

She paused to think that over, then said, "What were we talking about?"

That's when I started laughing and she started laughing. It's always the same.

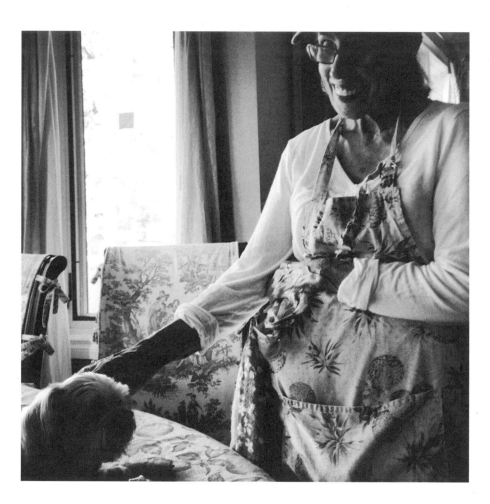

love it when mom smiles

Sometimes they will both be on the phone in different rooms and things really get interesting. More often than not they'll be talking to each other and I just go along for the ride. I treasure these crazy calls. I feel like I am in some kind of cosmic farce, watching them enjoy each other—one of the secrets to a marriage that has lasted almost six decades.

Good lord. That is something I will *never* experience, which makes me kind of sad. Unless I get married tonight and try to stay alive until I am 112 years old. Um . . . not gonna happen.

## November 15, 2014

Yesterday, my dad turned seventy-nine. I told him I couldn't believe he was almost eighty! He said that he still felt like he was a kid. "When I look in the mirror I just see me like I always was. I look the same as I ever did."

He doesn't have one single grey hair on his head and not too many wrinkles either. My mom says it's because of all the rum he drank—it "preserved" him.

I thought about what he said for much of the night. It's only when you see old pictures of yourself that you realize how different you look. I think I feel stranger about the person I used to be than the version of myself that I am today. I always think how sad it was that I actually thought I looked fat in old pictures when I was *so thin*!

Time trickles by and you see your face every single day and seldom do you notice the small and constant changes. I don't anyway. Although I did just spot a wrinkle by my nose that I'd never noticed before. . . .

There is so much grace in even being able to grow old. Sure, getting old is difficult, but *not* getting old is more difficult still.

Last night I had my parents over to my house, along with my little brother and his family, to celebrate Dad's big day. Dad seemed very unmoved by the whole thing. He said, "What's so different about today? We eat over here every day, so I guess every day is my birthday . . . ?"

Good point. Every day *is* your birthday. I have never been much of a birthday person, because much like my father, I feel like every single day I am here is a reason to celebrate.

I made pizza, because that's what Dad wanted, and a giant salad just to bring a sense of "we are eating healthy" to the get-together. Patrick and Jodi brought some very evil yet delicious cupcakes that were mostly buttercream icing. My mom LOVED them. We also had mini "turtle" cheesecakes that were a big hit. Dad, who has diabetes on top of everything else, had one of each, because "To heck with it, it's my birthday and I am going to be dead someday anyway."

My mom thought it was Pat's birthday most of the day, so we all had a good laugh about that.

After dinner we all sang a bad version of "Happy Birthday" and Dad sang along too, which was classic. These times are good ones. I keep trying to lock the memories away somewhere safe, so the "me" of the future will remember and smile.

# FOOLPROOF
# "TESTED A THOUSAND TIMES"
# PIZZA DOUGH

2 tsp fast-rising yeast (or one packet, if that's what you've got on hand)

1 ½ tsp sugar

1 generous cup very warm water

¼ cup olive oil

3 cups all-purpose flour

1 tsp salt

**I used to do this by hand, but now I use my KitchenAid with the dough hook. Doing it by hand works just as well, but needs elbow grease and some patience.**

Combine your yeast, sugar, warm water and olive oil in a large measuring cup. Stir gently and set aside. Put your flour and salt into a large mixing bowl and stir well.

When your yeast has activated (a few bubbles on the surface), add it gradually to your flour as you mix it on a slow setting. Make sure it's not too wet—you want the flour mixture to be able to form a ball and NOT stick to the sides. Same goes if you're mixing by hand. Add a little more flour if you need to.

Then I leave my mixer on knead for 7 or 8 minutes. Remove the dough and set on a well-floured surface. Shape the dough into a ball and knead a few more times. (Or knead by hand on a well-floured surface until the dough feels springy.) Cover with a clean tea towel and leave it for an hour to rise. It's now ready to roll out and use!

Put it on your pan, cover it with a little tomato sauce and your favourite toppings, and bake at 450 for 15 minutes.

Extra!

You can also use this dough to make naan bread. Pull off a small ball of dough. Roll it as thin as you can and fry it in a hot frying pan. I use spray oil directly on the piece of dough and I sprinkle it with a bit of salt. Flip it when you see the dough bubble up—it will only take a minute on each side, if that.

*mom and dad with leftovers*

# November 28, 2014

There's been a bit of a reprieve around here as far as my parents go. Everyone is sleeping well and eating well and enjoying the days. The TV remote has worked flawlessly for nearly a month. Nothing has been misplaced or picked up and carried off by the "movers." Everyone has their glasses, the credit cards are in Mom's wallet right where they should be, the dryer door hasn't mysteriously locked itself for no reason whatsoever. No one has fallen in the yard or wandered down the road or forgotten anything of any great importance.

It's funny how everything seems to ebb and flow, like a tide coming in and going out. Mom and Dad have these lovely conversations that float back and forth between them. It's like little birds fly out of their mouths with messages. They have been puttering around the house, putting a few Christmas things up in the yard, hanging the odd picture, cleaning our closets, pausing for cups of tea and toast slathered with thick sweet honey. It's like we've all slipped back in time about ten years.

I stand at their front door and see life as it was a decade ago and want to burst into tears. It's like Mom and Dad have been given a gift, a pause if you will, in what has been an otherwise exhausting series of crazy events. (For me, not them!)

I saw Mom this morning out in the yard wrapped in layers of coats and hats and scarves feeding the birds. A few days ago she fed them a tray of old cinnamon buns and some cheddar cheese. She is still tying strips of cloth in the branches for the squirrels and all the strips are gone in the morning. Thanks to my mom there are a lot of posh squirrel houses out there in the trees this winter.

I am making us a vat of pea soup for supper tonight and we have the latest installment of the Stallone franchise to watch. No clue what it's called, just that it's got every aging action star from the last four decades in it and my dad will love it.

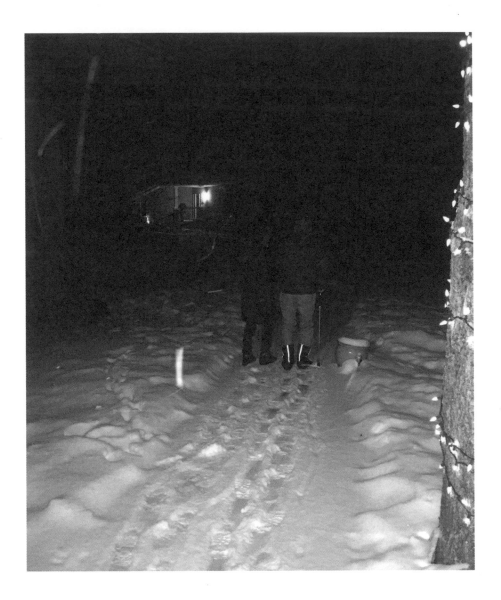

And my mom will probably nod off. We usually have to pause once or twice for a bathroom break (usually for me, not them).

Whatever this break is, whatever this delicate in-between stage may be, it has me shaking my head in wonder. Perhaps we get a little reminder every now and again of how good things were and can be, just so we can hang in there a little bit longer and don't end up completely mad at God. Or maybe not. Anyway, it's like a pre-Christmas miracle.

The cliché is that we are supposed to live our lives in "gratitude." But gratitude is not something you acquire like a Happy Meal from McDonald's. It's something you have to slowly create in your daily life through intention and sincere acts of goodness and kindness.

You can *say* you're grateful, but are you really? I don't ever use the word lightly. I have realized over the course of my life that gratitude has become the foundation of everything I do and everything I think. It's become a very tangible, tactile force in my music as well.

I do not get out of my bed without taking a moment to whisper, "Thank you." I can't go without saying it or my day loses some of its value.

Bear with me. Gratitude is a way to belong to the universe, a way to attach yourself to everything that ever existed. When grace and thanks and mercy fill your days, you can survive all hardship. You can conquer any wrongs, and you can help others to do the same. Gratitude is my cape, my superhero "must-have" to get me through life. Gratitude helps me to understand my parents and my shortcomings and my failures and my triumphs.

It has changed who I am and how I react to things. Without this magical energy in my life, I feel lost. There have been times when I didn't understand how much I took things for granted, and my whole being felt the effects of that negativity. I do not want to walk into the sunset anymore, I want to run into the sunrise. I am filled to the brim with gratitude.

# SPLIT PEA SOUP

¼ cup olive oil

1 smoked ham hock (ask your butcher)

1 large white onion, chopped

1 tsp cinnamon

1 tsp garam masala

¼ tsp cayenne pepper

salt and pepper, to taste

2 cups split green peas, rinsed well

8 cups (2 L) chicken stock

You can completely do this vegan too—screw the ham hock and use veggie stock and a few splashes of liquid smoke. If you don't have stock, you can just use water (though if you're using the water it tastes better if you have the ham hock).

Set a soup pot over medium heat. Drizzle in the olive oil, toss in the ham hock and onion. Add cinnamon, garam masala, cayenne, salt and pepper. (I use about a teaspoon and a half of salt to start but end up adding more to taste before I serve it.) Sauté the onion and the ham hock, getting a good sear on the ham, cooking until the onion is softened. This usually takes me 7 or 8 minutes. Add the stock and an equal amount of water—about 4 litres of liquid in total.

You're going to simmer this stuff for at least 2 hours. When the ham is falling off the bone, take the entire thing out of the pot and cut all the meat off into little pieces. Chuck the bone in the garbage and put all the chunks of ham back into the pot with your rinsed peas.

Simmer for another 45 minutes until peas are soft.

You're just about done.

At this point I take a hand blender and blitz it in the pot 5 or 6 times to break some of the peas into a paste, which naturally thickens the soup. You can also take about a cup of the soup and pulse it in a blender and then pour it back in the pot if you don't have a small hand blender.

Taste your soup.

You may need a bit more salt, you may need a bit more cayenne, you may even need a bit more cinnamon . . . taste it! Easier to add than take away. Making things too salty sucks.

# December 4, 2014

How do *you* feel?

It's hard being a person. The constant barrage of horrific and disturbing and sad and tragic news stories that pop up in front of our faces on our screens is nothing short of overwhelming. We are challenged on every possible level, our emotions tossed from side to side as though we were on a broken little ship lost at sea.

There are days where I find myself sitting in a chair, just trying to articulate *how* I feel. What do I feel right this second? What makes me happy? How am I going to get through the day while keeping my fragile sanity intact? Sometimes I just do not know how I feel.

My mom tells me that it's hard to negotiate the world these days even if you're sane. But how do you do it if you're somewhere on the cusp of sanity? We are all slightly broken. Some of us even rattle when we walk, and God forbid we should ever break into a canter—we'd sound like we were running open-armed through a china shop, knocking over every cup and every saucer and every lovely crystal dancing figurine.

Life blasts at us in billions of images every few minutes and we are expected to sort them all out and put them in their appropriate place in our hearts and heads. I wonder how most of us stay upright, to tell you the truth.

The pettiness of social media astounds me. I have been witness to the crushing wrath of the mob on many occasions over these past few years, seen people tossed away like they were a bit of old newspaper. It's sad that we sit here behind these keyboards and judge others with absolutely no regard to what happens to them afterwards. Victims of sexual violence come to mind. So many women are subjected to shallow and cruel jabs from other human beings who have never even met them, who have no facts to hand, save for the "facts" they have read on the internet, and yet feel compelled to spew their garbage at anybody who will listen.

How women breastfeed their babies, how they dress their dogs, how they dress for a party, what they wear to work, how much they weigh, what their legs look like in a bathing suit, how much cellulite they have, how they raise their children, how they vote, speak, look, act, smell—you name it, and we are there with a quick thumbs-up or a thumbs-down, making damn sure they know how very wrong they are. The insults pass back and forth like a pot of cold mashed potatoes at a really bad dinner party.

There are those that argue that the effect of social media is positive and useful and helpful and you can meet new friends and learn new things and you can "like" a dog or cat rescue, or join forces to ban Abercrombie & Fitch because they don't sell a size 12, or boycott the Russians. There is no end to it, and it's all . . .

exhausting.

Words are big. They define who you are. They are permanent. I don't think most people realize that. What you say is who you are. So try to be gentle on social media. Lift others up when you can, even if you don't agree with what they have to say. Don't always turn your words into weapons when you can just as easily make them doves.

# December 7, 2014

My dad wants to come over here earlier and earlier to have dinner. He called me at ten in the morning and asked me when would be a good time to come.

"Well, at suppertime, Dad."

"How many hours away is that?"

I could hear Mom in the background telling him that he had just had breakfast, for God's sake.

"Today it'll be about seven." I know I sounded, well, kind of curt.

"That's a long goddamn time to wait. Okay, then." I could hear how disappointed he was, and felt bad one more time about seeming so mean.

A while ago he rang my doorbell at 6:15 a.m. I was still sound asleep and at the shrill DING DONG I shot out of bed like a rocket. As I stumbled to the door I was cursing the moron who actually thought it was okay to ring somebody's doorbell at that hour. I threw open the front door thinking I would see one of the landscaping guys who had been putting in sod that week, but it was Dad standing there looking like he'd been up for hours.

"What's for lunch?" he asked and as he was clearly about to come right in, I got out of his way. I was grumpy, of course, but I managed to find the grace to follow him into the kitchen where I ended up making him a grilled cheese sandwich. He didn't talk to me, just sat at one of my stools and watched me make the sandwich. "Want a glass of milk?" I asked, and he nodded yes.

There is something about feeding people you care about that is extremely comforting for both of you. My dad looked six years old sitting there at my counter, his uncombed hair falling over his forehead. He has a hard time keeping still. It's like he has things to do but he doesn't know what those things are. Time to him is just a big mess and there is nothing for us to do but give in.

Despite the complaining I seem to do, I love seeing Mom and Dad coming toward my house at night to have dinner. Mom will call me to make sure it's the right time, usually more than once. They sit at the same spot at the table and wait for me to set their food down in front of them. They both look relieved to NOT have to worry about what to make themselves.

I hadn't planned on feeling the joy that I feel. I hadn't counted on the sense of well-being and accomplishment. The comfort I get from cooking simple food for my parents has come as a lovely surprise.

Here's a meal they both really liked:

# SHRIMP OR FISH TACOS
# WITH ASIAN SLAW

**SHRIMP:**

25 or 30 peeled and deveined raw shrimp

3 tbsp soy sauce

3 tbsp sweet chili sauce

1 tsp sesame oil

2 garlic cloves, crushed

**SLAW:**

1 pkg shredded coleslaw mix

a handful of cilantro (some people hate cilantro and if you're one of them use parsley or even basil)

3 green onions, chopped

¼ cup salted peanuts

1 red pepper, thinly sliced

1 carrot, shredded (I like extra carrot; usually the pre-made slaw mix has some in there)

**DRESSING:**

¼ cup olive oil

¼ cup rice wine vinegar

¼ cup soy sauce

splash of sesame oil

juice of 1 lime

½ tsp salt

½ tsp pepper

pinch cayenne

1 pkg corn tortillas

This seems like a lot of steps, but it's super easy to do. Honestly, I don't have the time to chop the cabbage for the slaw—I want fast and easy!

Put the shrimp in a bowl with all the marinade ingredients and refrigerate for at least an hour.

Put all your slaw ingredients into a big bowl. Mix or shake the dressing ingredients together and pour it over the slaw. You'll need lots of room to mix in the dressing—it can be messy! Put it in the fridge to chill.

Set a frying pan over medium heat. Throw in your shrimp, marinade and all, and cook until the shrimp are a solid pink colour.

Take out your tortillas and heat them up in the oven for a few minutes, or in a frying pan like I do—a little nonstick spray does the trick for easy flipping. Take 3 or 4 shrimp and put them in your tortilla, top with some slaw, fold and eat. Simple and good. . . .

# December 20, 2014

This year my mom didn't bring her Christmas tree up from the basement.

For the past decade, when the season was over, she has simply been draping the fully decorated tree with a giant bedsheet and having it carefully carried downstairs and stored in the corner. It suddenly seemed crazy to her to take all the decorations off every year, only to put them on again twelve short months later. "All Dad has to do," she said, "is plug the damn thing in."

When I asked her why she wasn't bringing it up this year, she just said that she didn't feel like it.

I guess Christmas the way it used to be—the way I remember it—is finally over. I have been having the dinner at my place for the past five or six years, but Mom had always taken the time to at least decorate her house.

She has a little village with street lamps and a church and a preacher and a snowman that all lights up. When I was young I loved looking at it for hours. She'd put it up on the mantel over the fireplace, just out of reach of our reckless fingers. It's sitting in its cardboard box now and I doubt it will ever see the light of day again.

The last year that Mom and Dad hosted Christmas dinner at their place was a few months after my dad had had a fairly major stroke. (He's had several small ones since.) He had got up at three in the morning and put the turkey in the oven, having stuffed it with a loaf of bread still in its plastic bag. He had sprinkled some kind of spice on it, which we never did identify, and cranked the whole thing up to 475 degrees. My mom smelled something in the night and jumped out of bed to find the turkey burning.

Dad had looked at her with such defeat and shame. On some level, he understood that he'd screwed up and done something that didn't produce the results he had hoped for—which was making us all a Christmas dinner, just like he had for the past forty years.

Later that day, we made a game out of guessing what Dad had liberally spread all over that poor turkey and had a good laugh. Dad said, "Pepper . . . lots and lots of pepper I think . . ." and then he laughed too.

This whole entire thing is about love and understanding and failing and getting up and trying over and over and over again to be the best version of ourselves we can be.

# December 24, 2014

Another year went slipping past us like a raindrop down a window. I remember on this exact day last year I was sitting right where I am now, reflecting on the previous 365 days of life's adventures.

Life ain't for the faint of heart. You have to wake up each and every day and realize that you can and will begin again. It doesn't matter if you've screwed up or lost your way or made giant mistakes or failed or fallen, you can always keep going forward.

You're not supposed to get it right out of the gate. My favourite people in the world, my dearest friends, all rattle when you give them a shake. They have little pieces that have broken off inside of them that are a constant reminder to them, and me, of how far they've come and how much they've learned and what they have survived.

The human spirit is unstoppable. You are an intricate part of everything that has ever existed or ever will exist and *that* is fucking fantastic. No matter what else is going on.

I guess Christmas the way it used to be—

the way I remember it—is finally over.

# December 26, 2014

Small changes gather speed and weight, then join together and get big without you really noticing it happening. And then you're faced with something like making the *entire* Christmas dinner at your house.

I mean, I'd been asked to bring a salad or a casserole, but never the whole turkey dinner—stuffing, gravy and all. But when Mom and Dad couldn't manage a big family dinner anymore—it was too confusing and far too complicated for two people who were both well into their respective battles with memory loss—I had to step up.

I remember the last Christmas dinner my parents attempted to put together. Dad was still able to drive back then, and they had picked up groceries, which they both loved to do. They bought all the things that one would need for a holiday feast. And there were still plenty of carrots and potatoes and onions from the garden— thank God, because that year we needed them.

Everything seemed to be in pretty good shape except that my parents had bought a five-pound turkey for fourteen people. I didn't even know turkeys could be that small. It was Christmas Day and there wasn't anywhere we could buy another bird. Dad looked as though he was going to sob and I did my best to tell him that everything was going to be fine.

I called my brother and told him to bring a ham and I peeled another pot of potatoes. I figured everybody could have a small piece of turkey, a slice of ham, and two pounds of potatoes and carrots.

We didn't have any stuffing, but we did manage to have a whole lotta laughs. I think that was the same year Mom made her famous cheesecake and we had to eat it out of bowls because it NEVER set. We laughed our heads off eating liquid cheesecake.

# January 7, 2015

I had a breakthrough of sorts a few days ago, right after I had a mini break*down*.

I'd asked my mom if she thought she would ever forget me and she said, "Well, my brain might, but my heart won't." Those eight words took my breath away. I felt a weight lift off my shoulders that I'd been carrying for the past few years.

It got me thinking about technology, oddly enough. I sat in my old red leather chair, right by the window overlooking my cluttered deck. It was strewn with shells from the peanuts the squirrels and the blue jays have made quick work of since November (I need to clean them up . . . I am becoming my mother, ever so slowly). The sun was streaming through the snow-covered spruce trees as if the beams were gliding in along a ruler, and I marvelled at their perfect geometry. But I digress. I was thinking about the "Cloud"—the Cloud that we are forever upgrading and meticulously monitoring to make sure all our files and pictures and contacts and *stuff* are kept safe and sound so we can find them again and look at them and remember.

Every thought we think, every memory we keep, every fond moment we experience and so eloquently recall as we forge our way through life, is important. They define who we are and why we are and where we've been. Our thoughts, our experiences, are what make us. Having said that, as I watch my parents lose those precious pieces of themselves, I wonder where those lost memories go. Surely they go somewhere?

I want to believe there is a celestial Cloud, hanging like a fly strip in God's porch, collecting every single thing we have ever done or said or thought or seen or heard or tasted. It's all there, stuck to that strip for eternity. We never lose it. It's saved forever. *We* are "saved."

My mom and my dad, and your mom and dad, and every other beloved person, dog and cat and bird and creature—they are all safe and sound and intact. What is forgotten here on earth will be saved.

Always.

# January 28, 2015

I have had many days in my life where my room felt like an ocean and my bed nothing more than a tiny ship being tossed around in complete nothingness.

I have experienced hundreds of hours in various states of worry and anxiety and hopelessness and doubt and fear.

All of this anxiety and depression is part of being a person. There is nothing more valuable to a human soul than time spent going through one's own mind and evaluating this thing called life. You're not supposed to be happy every waking moment of every single day. You're not a one-dimensional static entity—you are a constantly moving, evolving, growing, expanding body of energy. There will always be growing pains. Our souls are forever outgrowing our physical bodies, and it hurts our hearts and heads. It's bound to. Or we're stuck, and that hurts in a different way.

Depression can be managed. It can be put in a safe place, enabling a person to go forward with grace and even joy. It has to be managed, though, and that's the tricky part. You have to keep the lines of communication open with friends and family and professional helpers. Isolating yourself can be counterproductive.

Yes, it's great to be alone in order to dive deep into who you are and what makes you tick, but we are social beings. We need each other. We need that connection and that feeling of belonging, even if it's a few hours a week.

"Hope is the thing with feathers . . ." said Emily Dickinson. Feathers are the best flyers in the whole wide world.

I got myself up and out of my funk by making comfort soup. Enough for my folks to take home and have for lunch the next day.

# PULLED CHICKEN NOODLE SOUP

1 heaping tsp coconut oil or olive oil

1 medium onion, diced

3 medium carrots, diced

3 celery stalks, diced

3 or more garlic cloves, peeled and sliced (I use an entire bulb but I don't want to ruin your relationship)

1 tbsp salt, or to taste

1 tsp ground black pepper

¼ tsp cayenne

¼ tsp cinnamon

2 cups chopped cooked chicken—I like using some white and some dark meat

12 cups (3 L) water or chicken stock

a handful of fresh parsley

2 green onions, finely chopped

½ cup small dry pasta— small shells, alphabet or broken spaghetti

Any kind of chicken you want to use will work—barbecued, grilled, baked, boiled, a rotisserie chicken from wherever— whatever you have. Coconut oil is supposed to help with memory so I use that stuff on everything for Mom—I even "butter" her toast with it.

Put the coconut oil in a soup pot over medium heat. Add your onion, carrots, celery, garlic, salt, pepper, cayenne and cinnamon. Cook for a few minutes to soften your veggies, then add the chicken. I like using some dark and white meat. I usually cook this mixture together for 5 or 6 minutes to get some caramelization going.

Add your water or stock and simmer for 30 minutes. Add the dry pasta and simmer another 10 minutes, or until the pasta is cooked. Add the green onion and parsley and season with more salt and pepper if it needs it.

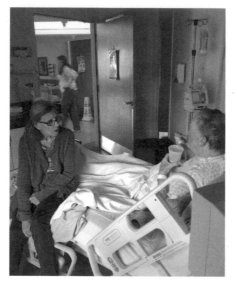

I am not even sure where to start. In a very short eight weeks, *everything* has changed. I haven't slept in days. This has been the hardest thing I have ever been through, no contest, and that includes a couple of severe heartbreaks and monumental personal failures of every kind.

Okay, so here's what happened. My dad had a heart attack five days after I left for a five-week tour. From the hospital, sadly, he went directly into a long-term care facility in Calgary. My mom's memory has failed so badly and his medical issues are so numerous that we simply could not keep him at home. The long list of what we've been dealing with: dementia, diabetes, kidney failure, heart failure, mobility, incontinence and high blood pressure.

Before I left, I'd hired a full-time companion to help my parents with the basics. Even though they had their own unique coping skills, their own unique dance, they were sliding into unsafe territory. With me gone, I knew they'd need extra help with meals and driving (Mom lost her licence three weeks before the tour was to start), laundry, simple organization and so on. Then Dad was taken to the hospital and my mom began a rapid mental decline. Removing him from her life's equation brought her house of cards tumbling down.

He was her everything. Even though she was the caregiver, he was her lifeline. She hasn't danced alone in fifty-eight years and it must be completely traumatizing to have had all of these sudden changes in every aspect of her life. It has been remarkable and frightening and fascinating to observe. I feel like I am standing on a sandbar in a strong current where nothing is certain, nothing is static, nothing is normal. I haven't cried at all, which is surprising. I feel like I am so busy trying to put the cards back into place that I haven't had the time.

My mom, always so strong and steady, sits sobbing into her tiny hands. She is filled with what looks to me like pure terror. She resents the fact that I had to have someone come to stay with her. No, she *hates* it. I am completely torn. She can't be alone anymore and I can't be there all the time. I thought she would like the help and the company, but she doesn't. Not at all. I pray that changes.

I hope we find our new normal soon. I hope that the sea we have been thrown into calms a little so we can reinvent ourselves. This is hard, but this really is life. And even a battered, hopeless spirit can find a way to keep going.

I think Mom will rally. I think Dad will be okay away from home. I am relieved that he has twenty-four-hour care, and that he is safe. We plan on bringing him home a few nights a week once he gets settled. I am taking him a bunch of little things this afternoon—throw blankets and an extra pillow, tissues and toothpaste and soap and salt-and-pepper Kettle potato chips as per his request. Some things never change.

I told Mom this morning that I was so sorry that she was sad and that I wished I could do more. She looked up at me and said, "Sad? What was I sad about?"

You just have to stay in such a moment and let it seep into every pore. Onward.

## March 27, 2015

I am taking my mom to Germany with me tomorrow. I have a job there next week, which I am so grateful for, and the company I am working with was gracious enough to let me bring Mom along with me. I cannot fathom being separated from your partner of fifty-eight years and learning how to be a new version of yourself. My mom told me it is like "little deaths" every day. Made my throat pinch ever so tightly. But she is forging on.

She was feeding the birds yesterday in her nightgown, apron, and giant down-filled winter coat that had belonged to her dad.

"That's quite the outfit you're wearing, Mom," I said.

She laughed. "I don't give a crap what I look like . . ."

And that made me laugh. Why should she care? I am twenty-six years younger than she is and I don't care anymore either. At some point, you have to claim your life and cast all doubt aside. It's simply too hard pleasing anybody else.

Today I thanked my mom for having me. She asked me why I was thanking her and I said, "Because you were giving birth to me fifty-three years ago and you said that I almost killed you."

"Well, you did almost kill me, but that's okay. We survived."

We did survive, and then some. She told me my head was so pointed from being "stuck" in there that she kept a hat on me for a year.

That's my mom. She pushed me out into the world and dared me to succeed. She gave me her bravery, for sure.

# April 7, 2015

It's never easy watching someone you love slip inch by inch down the rabbit hole. The more I think about it, the more sense it makes to me that Mom and Dad would come unravelled at the same time. They did everything together, and this trip into the unknown is no different. Even though they are physically apart, they will go towards whatever it is, hands clasped. It's their journey and all I can do is try to comfort them along the way. I can't save them from it, that's for sure.

The German river cruise with my mother was a gift, although she thought we were on a train trip. Since we could see the shore blur past us, I guess she assumed we were rolling along on tracks. I corrected her once and then caught myself when she was talking about it again: why do I need to tell her where she is and what she is on? I have to stop being the memory police, stop needing to be right all the time. It's exhausting and completely selfish.

I am going to make her one of those personal photo book thingies she can flip through to remind her of our first-ever trip alone together (unless you count the time we drove to Cranbrook for my brother's murder trial twenty-three years ago—but I digress). This trip was a hell of a lot more pleasant than that one.

The first night on the ship, I lay there in my little single bed and watched her across the room breathing in the dim light. She looked nine years old. I felt tears rolling down my temples and sliding slowly into my ears, making everything sound round and numb.

She said my dad's name out loud in the dark, several times, asking him to come to bed. "Derrel, Derrel, come to bed." It was haunting and life-affirming all at the same time. It took me hours to fall asleep. I was waiting for her to whisper secrets. . . .

Every morning I would lay out her outfits and help her get ready. I had never done that in my life and it kind of scared me. She'd gaze at the clothes draped on the bed and say, "Is that what I am wearing, Jann?"

"Yes, why?"

"I was just wondering. Does that go together?" She pointed at the socks that were black with gold stripes. "That doesn't go together."

"Does it matter, Mom?"

"I like matching socks. . . ."

I changed them to white.

As she pulled them over her bony little feet she said, "It's hard being a mother, isn't it?"

I nodded and had to turn my back so she couldn't see my face curl up into a ball.

My mom was graceful with everyone, quick with a smile and an outstretched hand. I was so proud of her. She outwalked half the dames on those inland excursions to wine villages and castles, climbing steep and crooked stairs with ease, not even out of breath while women half her age had to stop midway up and huff and puff. She never once complained about the rain, either—well, maybe once. She was in awe of everything. In the moment at all times, because that's where she lives now. That's where I need to live.

Dad is managing in the care centre. He talks endlessly about coming home, and it just about kills me. We'll start bringing him home for suppers and sunny afternoons in the yard, but not just yet. They have advised us to wait a few more

weeks, until he's better settled. I can understand that. Anyway, we are inching forward.

Mom told me yesterday that summer seemed so short this year. I told her it hadn't come yet and that made her smile madly. "It hasn't?"

"No, it's supposed to be spring, but it snowed again."

"Well, see, there are some good things about losing your marbles. Here I thought we were in store for months of this lousy weather!"

She turned around with her bucket of peanuts and continued hiding them one by one up in the trees. She likes to give the squirrels a challenge.

# April 12, 2015

The care facility called me yesterday to tell me that Dad had tried to escape. "Not to worry," they said. "We caught him before he got to the road. We're going to keep a better eye on him."

Apparently he went out a back door and down the alley on a beeline for home. He can hardly walk, so I can only imagine what "beelining" looked like for him.

It doesn't surprise me. No matter how long he will be living at his new place, he will be trying to get back to us. It's heartbreaking and heartwarming all at the same time.

Mom said she fully expects to look out the window one day and see Dad coming through the gate. "He could make it out here, Jann, he's that determined."

All of us have some sort of homing device at the very centre of us. We want to go home, always home, back to where we belong. Life is about belonging for me. Belonging to something, belonging to someone, belonging somewhere. No matter where I go, no matter how far I am across the globe, I am pulled back by a giant elastic band that is wrapped around my body a million times. Home. I know that's how Dad feels. His elastic is constantly pulling at him.

It's weird not finding Dad in his chair when I walk over to their house. He sat in it so much his head practically wore a hole through it. The chair just sits there now like something lost. There is something creepy about a chair that belonged to *one* person being empty. I want to set it out in the trees where we can't see it, but I know my mother would have a fit. Even though she says she doesn't like looking at it, she still wants it there in the middle of the living room.

I keep reminding her that Dad won't be coming home to sleep anymore. I don't want to lie. I don't want to make up some story that will make her keep wishing for him. It's not right. I don't lie to my dad either. When he asks when he will be coming home, I tell him that he will come to spend the afternoon and have dinner, but never to sleep. I tell him that those days are over. I simply cannot lie. It's not fair on any level. People may disagree with me, but I can't do it.

Mom is doing a little better every day, so that's a relief. She has the big dogs sleeping in the kitchen every night now so they are in heaven. They make her feel safe. I figure they will slowly make their way upstairs to her bedroom. They are good dogs, though, and I don't know what we'd do without them.

Mom told me that she was pretty sure they'd just let the burglars through the front door and show them where all the treats are. That made me laugh. Without laughter, all is lost.

## April 24, 2015

I was talking to a friend of mine this morning about feeling like I had become orphaned because my parents couldn't continue on in their roles the way I wanted them to. I keep trying to drag the past forward, like some giant sack full of stones. I want them—I *need* them—to be who they were. I can hardly pull that sack behind me, but it doesn't stop me from trying.

You have to let it go. I know that. I have to let my parents become who they are going to become. I have to make it easier for them to go forward towards their own destinies. I cannot change what is going to happen to them.

Change is a hell of a thing. I have to find some sense of grace for myself and not be repeating old behaviours over and over again. This has been the toughest time in my life, for many reasons, but I am getting a lot better at crying my head off. I am getting a lot better about getting really mad and howling at the moon.

## May 18, 2015

I feel like I have been living someone else's life these past two months. I stare at the ceiling in the middle of the night (which I can't really see because it's pitch black in my bedroom) and wonder how everything changed so quickly. Just a few months ago my life was completely different and the change makes me profoundly sad. It hasn't just been my parents, but also a million other things that have shifted around in my life and left me with a feeling of helplessness.

Still, Mom and I and my cousin Tracy (who drove all the way from Lethbridge) went into town to see Dad yesterday at the care centre and he seemed better than he had in a long time. When we got there, Dad was just waking up from an afternoon nap and he looked like he had a squirrel on his head.

Mom, of course, had to comment on that. "Derrel, what did you do to your hair?" She also asked him where his tooth was. I told her that his tooth had been gone for ten years and she was gobsmacked.

We have had this same conversation several times. A few weeks ago it went like this:

"Where the heck is your tooth, Derrel?"

"It's been gone a long time, Mom," I said.

"Well, that couldn't be possible! Jann, I stared at that head for fifty-eight years and he had a tooth in that spot."

"Well, I am telling you that his tooth has been gone for at least a decade. Don't you remember him spitting water through that hole to impress us with how far it would go with a little effort?" I couldn't quite believe she didn't remember that classic move. It was really something to behold.

"No, I don't remember one single thing about him spitting water through a hole in his teeth."

Dad sat on his bed and watched us talking like he was at a tennis match. He hasn't asked me to take him home with us for over a month. It used to make me feel like crying. I felt so guilty. I still feel guilty. I think the decision to move him out of the house will always haunt me a little bit. I know it was the right thing to do but it doesn't make the ache in my heart any easier to deal with.

But after the initial shock and grief, my mother is doing better without him at home. Not having to look after him twenty-four hours a day has reduced her stress. Her memory hasn't gotten worse. She doesn't repeat herself as much and she is sleeping better and laughing more. She is eating better and seems a lot more herself.

She was going down with the ship, as it were, and now her daily life is so much more manageable. Even she says she is glad she isn't having to deal with him all day long, though she feels guilty too.

We still see Dad almost every day and his overall health has improved as well. Getting his meds on time and on a consistent basis has been big, as is having constant companionship and help with mobility.

We are slowly getting to know the interesting people who live there with him. Betty, who has rollers in her hair every second of the day, and who is forever looking for her room. The "where is my aunt and uncle" lady who repeats that question for hours on end. The other day Mom said to Dad and me as we passed by this lady's wheelchair, "Would it kill you two to be this poor woman's aunt and uncle?" Dad laughed out loud.

# EASY VERMICELLI BOWL

1 pkg vermicelli noodles,
thick or thin, entirely up
to you and what you
can find at your
grocery store

2 tbsp coconut oil

1 bunch broccolini or
broccoli, cut into 1-inch
pieces

2 celery stalks, cut into
chunks

15–20 snow peas

1 red pepper cut into
1-inch pieces

4 green onions, cut into
1 inch pieces

2 tbsp soy sauce

1 tsp sesame oil

salt and pepper

chili flakes or hot sauce
(optional)

½ cup peanuts,
chopped

2–3 green onions,
chopped

1 tbsp rice wine vinegar

**This is something Mom really likes me to whip together on nights when we get home late from seeing Dad. It's vegan, too. . . .**

Soak your noodles in hot water as per package instructions. They usually need 7 or 8 minutes to soften up.

Get a wok or large saucepan going over high heat. Add your coconut oil and ALL the veggies. Add the soy sauce and stir constantly for 3–4 minutes. You want them to be crunchy—not soft and without colour.

Add your sesame oil for the last minute, along with a little salt and pepper, and I personally like some chili flakes or hot sauce.

Drain the noodles and get yourself a bowl. Serve the noodles with the veggies on top with a handful of crunchy peanuts and some green onion. The very last thing I do is sprinkle it with some rice wine vinegar—I love the bite it provides.

# June 3, 2015

We brought Dad home for the first time on Monday. I talked to him the previous afternoon and told him to be ready to go in the morning. I also told him that I was going to make him mow the lawn when he got here and he laughed a little bit. He has lost a fair bit of weight, perhaps twenty pounds or more. It worries me, considering that according to the staff at the lodge, he doesn't ever miss a meal. Mom says he is "dwindling away." She is the only one I know who uses that word, other than my gram. *Dwindling.* Good one.

When he walked through my front door he started to cry, which made my throat shut immediately. He seemed overwhelmed by everything. He kept saying that it all seemed changed and different.

 He can hardly walk now. Between the dementia and the blockages in his legs, he can maybe stumble a few yards at a time. We all grabbed an arm and an elbow and guided him over to the kitchen table. He wanted a Coke and his cup of coffee, which he had brought with him. He tried to talk but didn't really manage to get much out. He just blinked ever so slowly and looked carefully at our faces. I wondered what he was thinking about.

He was very calm and reflective. Like he was somehow living in slow motion while the rest of us were stuck on fast forward. I wanted to slow down too. I wanted to crawl into his head and watch the movie he was watching. My mom sat beside him and kept looking at him like he was an apparition.

"Are you tired?" she asked him and he nodded yes. We put him on the couch and

Mom untied his shoes and set them beside him on the floor. That too, made my throat squeeze nearly shut. It's the smallest things that set me off. It's the tiniest details that make my heart swell up like it's been stung by a thousand bees. You realize that things don't matter. Not the chairs we're sitting on or the mugs we're drinking out of or the clothes hanging off our shoulders. None of it matters. My dad doesn't care about his things anymore and to tell you the truth, he never really did. The man owns two pairs of shoes. He used to laugh at Mom and me and tell us that we could only wear ONE pair at a time. My mom would tell him that that wasn't the point!

I could tell that he wanted to go "home" after he had his hot dog. I don't know how to feel about that. The idea of home changes for all of us I suppose. It's a place in the heart not on the map.

## June 21, 2015

Father's Day has always been a bit of a quandary for me. I find myself on this particular Father's Day both guilty and, sadly, indifferent. Lots of people will be spattering the internet with glowing "I love you, Dad" banners and reminiscing about the times their fathers took them to baseball games and on fishing trips and whipped up barbecues on sunlit decks, and all those wonderful things that dads do.

That was never my experience with my own dad. He was an alcoholic for most of my formative years. My strongest childhood memory of Dad is of him screaming at us. He was the worst kind of drunk, the kind who had to be right, and liked to intimidate everybody around him. If we didn't bow to his every whim, we suffered the consequences.

Thank God, he was hardly ever home, because when he was around he was angry, he was brooding and he was always looking for a fight. My older brother got the worst of it. My dad picked on him constantly and I don't know why even to this day. Dad has never talked about it. Since he stopped drinking he's held his past as far away from himself as possible. Some of us would call that denial. . . .

I didn't realize that we weren't really a "normal" family until I was about thirteen. Mom would warn us not to bring other kids home from school "just in case your dad shows up."

How she hung in there still defies reason. "I did it for you kids," she'll say now and then. "I don't regret it."

It's funny how the difficult things in life can force you to go in certain directions. Had I not been wanting to avoid his frequent wrath, I doubt I would have sequestered myself in the basement, where he never came, so I could learn how to play guitar. Music became my refuge, my safety zone, the place where nothing bad ever happened, the situation I could control.

Don't get me wrong—my dad taught me countless, invaluable lessons. He didn't take any crap from anybody and, believe me, that rubs off on a kid. I remember how people reacted to my dad when he was determined to get his way, whether it was demanding another cup of coffee in a diner or his money back on a pair of pants that didn't fit. To this day, I don't tolerate nonsense in my business life. I expect people to be fair and ethical and decent. Period. If they're anything but that, they won't be working with me.

Seeing my dad now, in his room in the care centre, a mere shadow of his former self, is very hard. The man I used to be afraid of is now a meek and mild, helpless child. I was thinking about how much resentment I have been carrying around and how much I don't want to still be carrying it. I want to let it all go. Maybe today I'll start. I dragged it with me because I thought I needed it to protect myself. Silly what our hearts and minds do to us.

Even though he had his own struggles and his own demons, my father provided for us always. Even though he battled depression and addiction and failure, he managed to teach us important things, like working hard, and not giving up, and being your own person. He always showed up to help the neighbours build fences or move furniture or dig postholes or round up a lost cow or pour concrete driveways. He never stopped working and he never stopped being hard on himself.

I didn't always like my dad, but deep down I have always loved him. It's hard being a person. When I glance back at him as I walk out the door after a visit, that love resonates like never before. So I guess it's not indifference.

## July 4, 2015

It's hard how much things shift in the course of a few days. One of the most difficult things for me to get my head around is how much my mom can change even over a few hours. She can seem very clear and very much herself and then in the blink of an eye, she is gone: the person I've known for so many years leaves the building. I find myself feeling very resentful and bitter about this. I don't know how else to describe it. I get angry. I feel like somebody broke into my heart and took my most precious thing. My mother.

I don't know if I am mad at her for leaving me to fend for myself, or if I am mad at myself for being an asshole. I have a hard time being patient and being understanding. I fight the urge every single day *not* to be the memory police and constantly correct her. I so badly want to be mindful of living where she lives now and not expecting her to be where I am. That is no longer possible, certainly not on a full-time basis.

I know that, and yet I fight it constantly. My mother has been such an incredibly positive presence in my life. She has shown me, rather than told me, how to be a

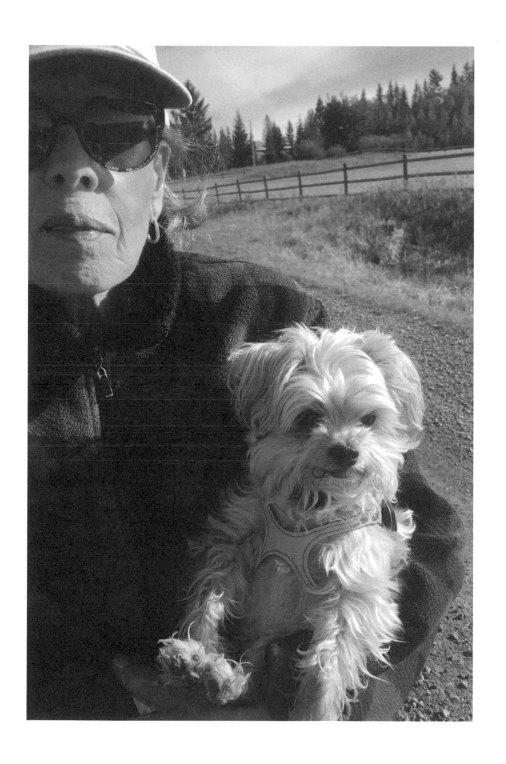

decent, empathetic human being. She's not overly sentimental or protective, but she's been a loving force behind me, whether I've succeeded or failed. I was an idiot over a period of many years. . . . I truly was. Some people say they have no regrets, but that isn't me. I have many. Yet my mother has always told me that I punished myself far more than she ever did, or would, and that is certainly true. She was the first person to ever tell me that I needed to learn to be kind to myself. When I was a kid, she rarely scolded me—she'd just have to look at me and I'd realize how far away from being my true self I was acting. I hated letting her down.

She worked full-time when my brothers and I were quite young, so making meals and doing chores were mandatory for us kids. I appreciate that so much now. As much as I *hated* helping around the house, I am so glad that she had the backbone to demand things from us. She expected us to show up for our own lives and to do good things. She was my mother and my mentor, *not* my friend. Friendship would come later, when I was old enough to appreciate what a friend truly is.

My mom still soldiers on through whatever life puts in her path. I have never heard her complain about anything, and I am not exaggerating. She doesn't complain. I have never heard her speak ill of another human being, either, except for my dad when he really deserved her wrath. I am in awe of her fortitude and steadfastness. She's fair and good and she can laugh at the worst of times. She has laughed us all through so much grief and loss.

But memory loss kicks everything and everyone around it in the balls, pretty much. The mother I knew is slowly going away. When she reappears, it's for shorter amounts of time. I feel alone and I want to blame somebody.

Right now she is losing track of what time it is, and getting up earlier and earlier. Sometimes she'll call me at six in the morning and ask me what I am doing and then she'll ask me what *she* is supposed to be doing.

"What do you want to do?" I ask, startled awake and with my heart pounding because I think something is terribly wrong.

"I don't have a clue," she answers cheerfully.

"Have you had coffee?"

"I think so. I can't seem to get over the time change."

"What time change, Mom?"

"I'm not sure . . . just the time change. I can't get used to it and I can't find my glasses."

"Did you check in your bed? You've been making your bed lately with your glasses still in it."

"Did I make my bed?"

And so we go, around and around, until I end up walking over to her house and finding her glasses and checking to see if the coffee is on and the bread is out on the counter.

"Did you have something to eat?"

"Yes, I did! I had some of that cake Deanne made me!"

She's so excited that she remembered she had cake, although Deanne is actually Nadine and I am actually the one who made her the cake. It's all I can do not to set her straight. It's all I can do to not sit at the kitchen table and bawl my head off.

# August 18, 2015

I haven't written anything in a long time. Life has a way of picking you up and dropping you off a few weeks later at an unknown destination. Some days it really does feel like I've been plunked down in a strange land surrounded by strange people and strange things I hardly recognize. My own house feels "funny" when I've been away for a while. Autumn is already nipping at the flowers and the grass is slowing down. Right now even a change of seasons is unsettling.

My dad is fading away. Literally—he's lost forty pounds in the past six months. The weight is falling off him like it wants to go somewhere else, anywhere but where his body has found itself. He looks at me like I have an answer to his quandary, when in fact, I do not. His unhappiness is palpable.

They moved him to a more aggressive dementia wing of the facility because he had become combative with the staff, verbally and physically. Now he's basically strapped to a wheelchair for the entire day. Before they started tying him in place, he'd struggle to get up then crash to the ground like gravity was his lover. It was bad. It was constant. He was injuring himself and they were concerned for his safety. I understand that. They told me they had no choice but to strap him down, but he is miserable.

I've been on the road for work these past few weeks and when I saw him today, it was shocking. His face has changed so much. It made my eyeballs hurt trying to keep the tears from shooting out like bullets. I know he's dying, an inch at a time. I can't tell you how helpless we all feel, watching him slither his way down into the earth. I pray at night that he will go to sleep and simply not wake up, but the world doesn't work that way.

I guess he still has work to do here on planet Earth. It doesn't make it any easier to think that God has a plan for my dad. It doesn't make the hurt and pain and angst and worry one little ounce less. Watching him go is hard, but that's what people do. They make their way out of this world the best way they can. One breath at a time.

## August 31, 2015

I am sitting in the Chicago airport. I'm trying to get home. Dad is barely hanging on. He was unresponsive when they rushed him to hospital. Pneumonia. Another little stroke. Low blood pressure and racing heart. The man is worn out.

My little brother, Patrick, has been with him night and day, along with Jodi. Dad's two sisters and his sister-in-law came up from Lethbridge to see him yesterday. Mom has been there, too. Pat and Jodi brought Mom to their house to sleep while I've been away.

Every damn time I go away that father of mine gets himself hauled off to a hospital. Perhaps he likes having me frantically trying to get home to him. Still, looking after Mom and Dad for these past five or six years is the best thing I've ever done. The lessons learned have been too many to count, and the value beyond priceless. Caring for people makes you better. Period.

I hope I get home in time to say goodbye, but if I don't I have a great sense of peace. I stopped being mad at him a long time ago. I started forgiving and I started letting go of all the things that didn't really matter in the long run anyway. Funny what finally makes you let all the hurt and anger go.

## August 31, 2015

With Dad now.

# August 31, 2015

Dad passed away at 8:15 p.m. We love you.

# September 1, 2015

Oh, what a day. I feel like I am tangled up with all these loose ends that life has decided to gather up and hand to me. Here, life says, untangle all these little puzzles and get back to me when you've figured it out.

Every thought in my head has a hundred layers. Layer upon layer of pain and confusion and disbelief. It's like the world decided to test how much chaos it could inject into my heart without it stopping. And my heart keeps going. The blood whirls around inside my chest like a tsunami, gathering up every memory and pushing them all out my tear ducts. I try to keep myself from crying and I don't know why. It actually, physically, hurts my jaw *not* to cry. I don't know why it's my jaw that hurts—that's just where the pain ends up.

People are buzzing around me, saying important things, and I nod and say things back to them like: "I don't think I have ever seen or heard anything so terrifying as my father gasping for air on that tiny bed. . . ." And then I wonder if I said it out loud or if I just said it in my head. I am pretty sure it was in my head because they are asking me how I am doing and I don't even know because I feel like I am on mute. I am adrift inside my breaking heart.

I kept telling him to go. I remember that.

I was thinking that it was taking so long, that he was working *so* hard to get out of himself. His struggle tore me and my little brother into shreds of something we couldn't even recognize.

I kept looking across the bed at Patrick and whispering, "Where is the peace? Where is the fucking peace?"

It never showed up.

Not until that last unusual moment.

A strange noise crept out of his lungs like it was embarrassed. Dad looked straight up and finally left his body there, in the blue-and-white cotton gown that had probably been worn by a hundred other sick and scared people.

I felt like I died too.

We all did.

I thought for a second that I felt him pull at my sleeve, but it was only my heart beating so hard that it was moving my arm up and down ever so slightly.

Part of me wishes I hadn't seen any of it, that I could have just remembered him walking away from my house, arm in arm with Mom, carrying their leftovers.

But I stayed in the thick air of that little "comfort" room for him.

Because I knew he was scared.

# September 17, 2015

It's been a couple of weeks since Dad went off on his new adventure through time and space. His wooden urn now sits on my kitchen counter, watching me walk around each morning with my hair hanging down. We haven't decided what to do with him. I think he is happy here, though, although he doesn't say it outright. . . .

I will tell you that it has felt like a storm pouring down emotions. One minute you're up and the next minute the discomfort is agonizing. Anxiety has tiny little teeth and they nip at you with great persistence. I can't describe the blanket of fear that folds itself over me at times. I can hardly breathe, and then it lifts like it was never there at all. Funny.

I wish I knew when it was coming, though, because I would lock the doors and close the windows. But I don't, and simply have to go through it. You can't skip the hard bits in life. I feel ridiculous even writing this, because what are my hard bits compared to the troubles going on in this world, the profoundly horrific things people face every single hour of the day: the war, the hunger, the violence, the loss, the hardship? My troubles are little invisible things that God doesn't have time for. Nor should he take the time . . . I know that. No matter what happens in my life, I am filled with gratitude.

Two days after Dad passed away, Mom was officially diagnosed with Alzheimer's. Her condition has been a blessing in a sense, as she has seemed to deal really well with everything. The disease somehow tempers sentiment, at least at this stage— that's what I have found anyway. Of course, she's very sad, but it's manageable. I think had he died four or five years ago, she would have been flat on her back with grief. She tells me she forgets to be sad. She is still somehow very funny, perhaps without knowing it.

For instance, when she and I drove home from the hospital after Dad had gone, it was very quiet and eerie in the car. We were both processing the hours and hours of his labour: death is much like a birth. At one point, Mom turned to me and said very calmly, "Well, I can't believe that you had him put to sleep, Jann." I just about drove off the road.

"Put to sleep? I didn't have him put to sleep, Mom!"

"I saw you give him that needle."

"I would never do that! It's illegal for starters."

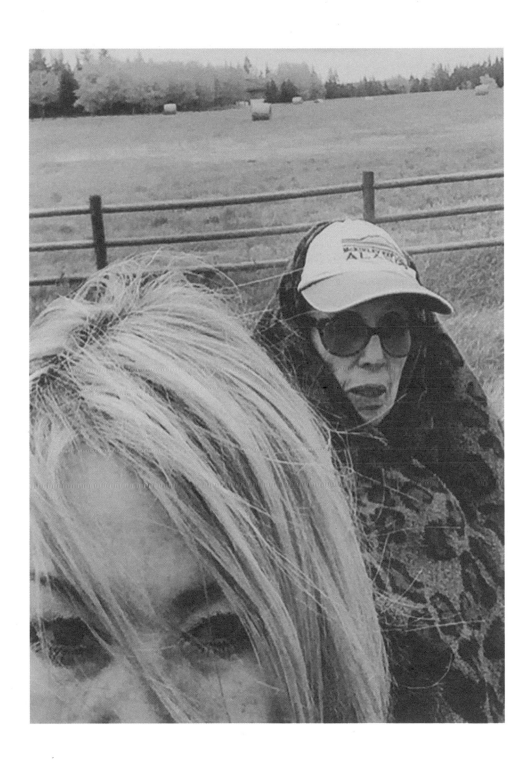

A few more minutes went by as I could feel her thinking hard about everything. Then she turned towards me and said, "Did Dad give you permission to have him put to sleep?" Her hands were folded on her lap, her fingers twisted like tight bits of rope.

"Mom, he died of complications from a lot of things. He was so worn out and tired and fed up . . ."

"I saw what I saw . . ." she said. She was convinced that I had him put down.

I wanted to laugh but it felt completely inappropriate. When I think of it now, though, it makes me smile. In all that sadness, the absurdity of what she was saying to me somehow erased the pain for a moment or two. I knew at that moment that we'd would stumble along somehow, and figure it out one small thing at a time

## October 8, 2015

My mom amazes me every single day.

## October 9, 2015

Anxiety is new to me. You'd think that after fifty-three years on the planet I'd be well past having new things happen to my body, but I guess I'm not. My own flesh seems to be in revolt against me.

One minute I'm sitting here minding my own business and the next minute this thing wraps my torso like a python and decides to squeeze the ever living hell out of my heart and suffocate me at the same time. It's beyond scary.

I kept thinking I was having your mid-life garden-variety heart attack. My instinct was to sprint around the house in full-on panic mode while attempting to dial 911 and then run out into the middle of the yard and start yelling for help while I was waiting for the ambulance to arrive. I didn't. The rational part of my brain kept reminding me not to believe what I was thinking and told me to stay put and keep breathing in and out. So that's what I did. I shut my eyes, concentrated on breathing in and out, and told myself I was okay . . . over and over again. I didn't expect it to work, but it did.

For the time being.

Anxiety doesn't stick to a schedule. It's its own boss and it's the worst boss I've ever had.

After that first assault, I was on full alert waiting for the python to come back when I least expected it—when I was walking through the mall or sitting on a plane thirty-eight thousand feet in the air or walking the dogs or eating soup or watching a movie. I was ready and waiting for something that may never happen again and that pissed me off. It pisses me off.

I have learned that anxiety loves it when you sit still and worry. It hates it when you engage with friends and laugh out loud and get fresh air and keep moving. It hates it when you don't give up and when you're creative and insistently filled with hope. Anxiety doesn't let go of you easily but that doesn't mean you can't be in the same room with it and still get stuff done.

# October 28, 2015

It's been two months since Dad died. I moved him in his little mahogany box to a spot in my living room. We are going to figure out where to lay him to rest in the spring. There were so many decisions to make when it first happened that we simply haven't gotten around to it yet. I think he likes it here in my house. Mom always says that she can't believe that they fit all of him in *there*—she points at the urn. I don't comment.

It's all still weird in a thousand different ways. I'm not really used to the idea of never seeing him again. Mom, however, says she sees him all the time.

"He was in the cupboard above the sink in the bathroom last night, Jann, and he looked SO young!"

"The cupboard?" I said, lifting an eyebrow.

"Yes. You don't believe me but he was there as plain as day. He looked really good."

"Does he say anything to you?"

"Not a word. He just looks at me for a while and then he disappears."

I love having these conversations with my mom. They make me happy from the inside out. I don't know if it's the Alzheimer's, but she sees him and it's as real as anything. I asked her if she was scared when he showed up. "Not one single bit," she said waving her hands through the air. "Why in the world would that scare me? We were married forever."

"Well, it would scare the living shit out of me, Mom!" And it would. I would run out the front door screaming if my dad showed up in my bathroom cabinet to stare at me.

Still, part of me is a little bit jealous that she is able to see him—and that she has such an open heart and mind that she's not the least bit freaked out by seeing a dead person in her bathroom. She says often that she just forgets to be scared. I need to forget to be scared too.

# November 22, 2015

I have my mom propped in her favourite chair watching a Western with Gregory Peck. She was agitated when she got here at 7 a.m., but she's settled down a bit. Her disease is stealing her sleep and her sense of reason and her sense of self. For the first time, I can see the paranoia slipping in and out of her mind like a thief, stealing memories.

We've spent the last few hours going around and around in a giant circle and I'm exhausted. My mom doesn't know she has Alzheimer's. How could she know? She doesn't know why I have the Christmas tree up. She asked me this morning if I needed help taking it down. I told her we hadn't had Christmas yet. She looks at me, perplexed, then tries to cover her tracks. Her mind is busy trying to hide its problem. The mind is so tricky. It constantly re-configures, rewires, reroutes, trying to protect itself from what it knows.

I can't imagine how maddening it must be for her. I mean, I get so anxious I feel like crying most of the time. The disease is taking me over too, even with the help I have. None of that changes the fact that I am losing my mom, an inch, a thought, a memory at a time.

She just told me she doesn't want "those ladies" in the house anymore—meaning the lovely souls who help me at night because Mom can't be alone. She says she doesn't need them because she is getting better. "I will beat this," she says. I just mumble, "Okay. I hope so, Mom." And then a few seconds later, she tells me that she hates being alone in the house.

"That's why the ladies come in the evening, Mom."

"Oh," she says, nodding. And around we go. . . .

I tell her that I love her more than anyone in the world and that I am making decisions for her that I know she would be making for me if I was in this shape.

"I am sick of you telling me I'm sick," she says sternly.

I tell her I am sorry.

Then she says, with a smile on her face, "Should we take the tree down?" She loves to be helpful.

"Why don't we leave it up for a while?"

"Until New Year's?"

"Sure, New Year's would be good."

"I wish you didn't have to go away all the time."

"Me too, but we all have to go to work."

"Maybe I'll retire . . ."

"I think you should retire. You've been working for fifty years."

"I have?"

I laugh, and we go back to the top of the same pile again. And then I make her my favourite pancakes.

# GUILT-FREE FLOURLESS BANANA-PEANUT-BUTTER-EGG PANCAKES WITH MAPLE SYRUP

2 eggs

1 banana

¼ cup peanut butter, or almond or cashew butter

pinch salt

**I love to eat these at least once a week!!**

Put all the ingredients into a blender and pulse until well mixed. It'll look like pancake batter, only a little thinner as it has NO flour.

Set a frying pan over medium heat and spray it well with nonstick spray, or they will stick. Pour the batter into small dollar-sized pancakes and cook for 30 or 40 seconds a side. (Don't make them very big or you won't be able to flip them. #truth)

This recipe usually makes about 20 pancakes. I smother them with butter and maple syrup. So does Mom.

# December 11, 2015

I feel like I'm making good decisions for us most days, but of course, there are times when I feel like I am completely lost in the fog. Mom now gets very anxious at some point during every day. Mostly in the mornings when she walks over to my place. She struggles with having "the homeless people sleeping on my couch every night . . ." She means the women I've hired to make sure she's never alone. Nadine and I have decided to order a "bed chair" for the office so the "homeless ladies" can nap in there, where she won't see them first thing when she wakes up. Mom told me this morning that she is doing her best to look after them, which made me want to bawl. Her heart is so big.

She also told me that she wanted to be normal again and I told her why in heaven's name would she want to be that? I told her normal was for the birds. That made her laugh. I am getting better at moving her away from an issue that she has fixated on. I talk about really abstract, fun things that distract her from thinking about her troubles. It has to be so difficult trying to make sense of everything that darts around her mind. I can't imagine. Perhaps one day I too will experience this dreaded thing, this loss of self.

Mom misses her independence more than anything. "I just want to walk down the bloody road and get the bloody mail, but I can't seem to do anything without those people trailing behind me," she says. She hasn't wandered off anywhere yet, but I expect that will be one of the things that will come eventually. We head back to the doctor on December 16 and I told Mom she could ask him any questions she might have about what's happening. I told her we could write them all down. "Fine," she said. "I've got a few things to tell that guy!"

We have lots of laughs every day, despite it all. Mom had a cataract operation last week and told me afterward that she didn't think that she and doctor saw "eye to eye." She can still be so witty.

I guess I assumed that at some point Alzheimer's people would know what was happening to them, but they don't. She doesn't, though she did tell me that I needed to get my brain checked too. I agreed.

It broke my heart today when she said, "I feel like I am sitting in this house waiting to die." I should take her somewhere in January, give her something to look forward to, even if she forgets what that something is.

I do feel sad a lot.

It's hard to lose your mom a bit at a time.

It's weird and frustrating.

Sometimes she is so there, and I cherish those moments. I hate seeing her cry. She'll tell me she doesn't even know why she's crying. I don't think it's important to always know why.

# December 20, 2015

My mom always wants to do something for me, to help in some small way. She never wants to be idle or just sit on the sidelines while life is going on around her. I hate to admit this, but from time to time I feel like I take advantage of the fact that Mom likes to mop and vacuum. I may have her run over my floors more often than they really need doing. . . .

But in my defence, it keeps her busy and more than that, it makes her *happy*. Mom still wants to have a purposeful life, to be wanted and useful. She can fold a basket of tea towels for an hour and not be the least bit bothered, in fact she'll tell me how much she enjoyed it. She loves wiping counters and watering plants. Although it's

very difficult for her to stay on task. She'll have a potato peeler in one hand and a potato in the other and still have to ask me what she's doing. Then she'll peel that potato down to a nubbin if I don't keep an eye on her. I usually have her stir a pot of soup if I have it going, or slice up an onion. Onions can be cut into any shape under the sun and they'll work just fine in a recipe.

I think she misses cooking a lot, because she wants to be in the kitchen as much she can. I am always trying to figure out what she can do without setting something on fire or cutting off one of her fingers. I am getting better at just letting go of details. Details don't matter. I'm the only one bothered that the tasks she does can be repetitive; she doesn't care how much she does any one thing.

I'm trying to help my mom feel as normal as possible, even if it's a bit uncomfortable for me. Being around food and helping to prepare it makes her feel like a regular person. She can peel a carrot for an hour for all I care now, whatever it takes to feel purposeful is what it's all about.

Tonight we have company coming, and she cut up all the onions for the finger food. We also served my favourite salmon and my favourite asparagus dish.

# CARAMELIZED ONION AND BLUE CHEESE PUFF PASTRY TART

1 pkg puff pastry, thawed

¼ cup olive oil

2 tbsp butter

2 white onions, thinly sliced (mild Spanish work the best)

2 cups sliced mushrooms—whatever you have on hand; use a variety if you like

½ cup sliced, pitted Kalamata olives

½ tsp salt

½ tsp pepper

pinch cayenne

1 cup grated Parmesan cheese

¼ cup crumbled blue cheese

3 tbsp balsamic vinegar

This makes great finger food when you cut it up in little hunks. Puff pastry is in the frozen food section of your grocery store. Do not buy phyllo pastry—it's an entirely different thing.

Make sure your puff pastry is completely thawed before you roll it out into a large rectangle that's about 10 inches by 14 inches. Don't worry what it looks like! Rustic is good—just make sure it's not thicker than ¼ inch. Line a cookie sheet with parchment paper and place your rolled-out pastry on it. Set it aside.

Set a deep-sided frying pan over medium heat and add the olive oil and butter. Add the onions, mushrooms and olives, get them cooking down and then add salt, pepper and cayenne. Sauté everything for 6 or 7 minutes, stirring constantly because it burns easily. Add the balsamic vinegar, stir well and cook for another minute or so. Remove from the heat and set aside to cool for 10 minutes.

Preheat your oven to 375°F. Poke the dough with a fork 6 or 7 times—this will keep it from bubbling up too much. Spread half of the Parmesan cheese on the dough, then the cooled mushroom, olive and onion mixture on top of that. Sprinkle with the rest of the Parmesan cheese and the blue cheese, spreading evenly.

Pop the tart into the oven for 35 minutes, or until golden brown. I can always tell by the sides of the dough how it's going—they should be a fairly dark golden brown colour.

Let cool for 10 minutes and then slice into squares.

# FRESH MOZZARELLA, GARLIC, OLIVE OIL AND SEA SALT ON TOASTED BAGUETTE

1 baguette, sliced into
½-inch slices on a
slight angle
2 garlic cloves, peeled
and left whole
sea salt
olive oil
fresh mozzarella

**These are so darn good—you'll eat 3 or 4 before your guests even get to your front door.**

Brush your slices of baguette lightly with olive oil and set them on a baking sheet.

Toast them under the broiler in your oven until evenly toasted. Keep your eye on them—it doesn't take long! I'm telling you this because I've burned them dozens of times! Do not do anything else. Watch the damn oven.

Remove the toasted baguette from the oven and immediately rub your garlic over each piece of baguette. I usually go through two whole cloves. ·

Rip the fresh mozzarella into chunks and put them on the toasts. You'll want them to look pretty uniform. Drizzle more of the olive oil over each piece and sprinkle with some sea salt.

# MAPLE AND GINGER SALMON
# WITH GREEN ONION

½ cup maple syrup (use the real stuff for crying out loud)

1 thumb-sized nub of fresh ginger, finely grated

½ tsp cayenne

1 tbsp coconut oil

4 3-oz salmon filets

salt and pepper

2 green onions, finely chopped

This is a good one to scale up or down, depending on how many you have coming for dinner. And again, it's so easy.

Preheat oven to 425°F.

In a bowl, mix together the maple syrup, ginger and cayenne. Set aside.

Set a big oven-proof skillet on the burner on medium high. Heat up the coconut oil in it. Sprinkle the filets with salt and pepper and lay them skin side down in the hot pan. DON'T FLIP THEM! Cook them for 2 to 3 minutes.

Remove from heat and pour over the maple syrup mixture. Bake in the oven for 10 minutes, until the glaze is slightly caramelized. Sprinkle with green onions and serve with white rice or a side salad.

# BLUE CHEESE AND
# ALMOND ASPARAGUS

1 big bunch asparagus (15–20 spears)

3 tbsp butter

¾ cup crumbled blue cheese

¼ cup slivered almonds

salt and pepper

A great side dish with pretty much any protein or pasta.

Blanch the asparagus until fork tender. I prefer them a little more on the firm side. Remove from water and set in a shallow casserole dish. Immediately cover with butter, blue cheese and almonds, and salt and pepper to taste.

# January 3, 2016

You died in the early evening on the last day of August, Mom's birthday—making extra sure we'd remember you on that date, year after year. Like we would ever forget you. I still struggle with you going the way you did. You were not the least bit peaceful, Dad. Not a single one of your last breaths came and went without a lot of effort on your part.

You didn't want to go. You said as much, dozens of times. You were afraid of dying and I don't want to be afraid like you. When death comes over the horizon to take me back to wherever I came from, I want to find some small thread of bravery hanging off my sleeve.

Your death was loud and raspy and the whole room seemed to be under water. None of us could breathe, either. You and your spirit filled every single corner with heaving booms. I thought my head was going to blow off. The pressure was massive. You were in my bones, Dad. I felt you pushing through my flesh like a bullet.

I'd never watched anybody die before and, sometimes, I wish I didn't have that memory of you in peril burned into the back of my retinas. I sometimes wish I had not been there at all . . . but then I catch myself. Patrick reminded me that we were there for *you*, to keep you company, to carry your fear for you.

But even so, you didn't find it easy to go. There's got to be a lot to do when at last the spirit separates from the body. Last little details that have to be attended to. Pacts made with God and the spiritual cleaning up that comes with having been on the planet for eighty years.

Years of diabetes and kidney failure and heart attacks and infections and strokes, and in the end you died of pneumonia.

Mom kept saying, "He's had it, Jann. He's tired. . . ."

She kept asking Patrick if the nurses could at least give you a cough drop. Pat looked at me and shook his head. "She doesn't know he's dying. . . ." he said.

"No, she doesn't," I said.

And then you went. You made a sound that I will never forget. It was part moan and part holler and part lament and part cry and part cheer.

Yes, a cheer.

Finally split apart from the 160-pound body that was keeping you from the abyss. From the wonder. From the glory of the unknown.

I should have stayed with your body longer, afterward, but I couldn't.

Pat pulled the covers up around your neck and kissed you on the forehead and we walked out into the bright lights of the busy hospital.

# February 27, 2016

I was so used to having Mom and Dad around, both emotionally and physically— they lived fifty feet from my door for nearly ten years. I have been able to hire enough help that Mom can stay in her house, which has been wonderful for her and me. But she can't be alone anymore and she hates it. *Hates* it. The Alzheimer's dilemma: stay in your own house, but have people there with you all the time, or go into full-time care and *never* be alone again. It's the only way I can get her to understand that we have to have the ladies around. It could be so much worse, I tell her. But Mom keeps saying she wants to be normal.

She can't be alone anymore and she hates it.

"What do you mean normal?" I ask her.

"Like other old people."

"Other old people are in nursing homes, Mom."

"No, they're not."

"Yes, they are."

"Not all of them are."

I tell her she has memory problems and that's why we need the help. I try to never use the word dementia, or Alzheimer's. I don't want to scare her. On some level she still thinks she is perfectly fine. I asked her what year it was. She told me it was 1912. That was the year her mother was born: a date cemented into her brain.

Who is our prime minister?

"That little twerp—the son of that other dead guy."

That made me laugh. She knows who it is, and I didn't need to hear the actual name.

What month is it?

"It's May," she says matter-of-factly.

"It's actually February."

"Good God, you mean we have *more* winter coming?"

"I'm afraid we do."

"Well, that's terrible."

"Tell me about it."

"Tell you about what?" she says, smiling. I realize she's kidding around with me.

We go back to the topic of the ladies in her house.

She thinks they are all homeless, and complains that one of them does laundry non-stop. I joked that maybe I should bring my dirty clothes over and she could wash them too while she was at it. Mom thought that was funny, though not super funny.

"I think she is doing an entire family's laundry, Jann."

"Well, at least she's clean."

"That's true," Mom says. "I couldn't have a dirty person in the house."

"You have a muddy dog in the house every day."

"I don't care. Belle's allowed to be whatever she wants."

"Don't you get tired of all the dog hair?"

"I don't notice it. I don't focus on those kinds of things. It's a waste of time."

Indeed.

## March 27, 2016

I'm sitting here with Mom, who is eating a giant piece of my birthday cake and drinking the last few slugs of her Budweiser. My pal Chris ordered me a gorgeous cake that was a work of art and I didn't even want to cut into it. But yeah, we *did* cut into it and then devoured the whole first tier. It's probably the closest I'll ever get to a wedding cake.

My little brother and sister-in-law took Mom to church this morning and she told me that it was "too religious" for her liking.

"But church is supposed to be religious and it's Easter after all."

"No, it's not supposed to be religious. It's supposed to be inspiring and uplifting with a positive message. This was just a bunch of nonsense. There were no songs and I didn't like the preacher."

"Did you have lunch in the basement afterwards?"

"No, because they've given a lot of people food poisoning."

"Damn nuns."

"There weren't any nuns." Mom shovelled another forkful of cake into her mouth. "They are just normal women."

"Damn normal women."

Humour is ALL.

Laugh at all the heartache.

Laugh at all the pain.

Laugh at all the silly things you thought you did in vain.

Laugh at all the guilt.

Laugh at all the wrong.

Laugh until you can't be anything but true and strong.

## May 8, 2016

I am so grateful as I sit here next to my sleeping mother. She is having a nap after a great visit with Patrick and Jodi and their twin boys, Ethan and Ryan. She had her beer early, and so she should: today is her day.

I'm grateful for all the times she dragged herself out of bed to drive us to our hockey practices and our baseball games and our basketball and volleyball and badminton tournaments.

For the thousands of Crock-Pot meals and countless words of encouragement, and for her limitless support no matter how badly we'd screwed up.

For telling me my arms were just right and my freckles were perfect and that I was sturdy and not the least bit fat.

For looking past my mistakes and seeing my potential.

For letting me fail.

For hoping for me when I couldn't seem to hope myself.

For sticking it out with Dad, even when it seemed so dismal and pointless. For picking us all up even when she was down.

For inspiring all of us with her determination and bravery.

I have a good mother, and her voice is still what keeps me here.

Feet on ground

heart in hand

facing forward

be yourself.

In honour of all those Crock-Pot dinners, here's my version.

# ROASTED ONE-POT
# WHOLE CHICKEN DINNER WITH
# SPUDS AND PEAS
# AND CARROTS AND ONIONS

1 large white onion (or whatever onion you happen to have on hand)

2 large carrots

2 potatoes

¼ cup olive oil (plus more as needed)

salt and pepper

pinch cayenne

1 roasting chicken (they are usually between 3 and 4 pounds)

2 tbsp seasoning salt (your fave)

3 whole garlic bulbs (yes, I mean the whole thing, not 3 cloves)

1 cup frozen peas (or fresh, if you have them)

**This could not be more straightforward.**

Preheat your oven to 425°F.

Cut up the carrots, onions and potatoes in medium-sized chunks. Put half of them in the bottom of the pot. Drizzle with olive oil, sprinkle with salt, pepper and cayenne. Plunk the chicken on top of the veggies. (I rinse the chicken and pat it dry because that's what Mom always did.)

Smother the bird with olive oil and rub in your seasoning salt and some pepper.

Stuff the rest of your veggies around the chicken, including the garlic with the tops of the bulbs cut off with a sharp knife. Don't slice your fingers off as I have done several times.

The pot I use belonged to my mom's mom—it's an oval ceramic pot that is stuffed to the hilt by the time I have everything in there. I can hardly get the lid on, so don't worry if you think your pot is too full.

Drizzle some more olive oil on the veggies and add a bit more salt, pepper and cayenne. Cover and put it in the oven for 45 minutes.

Don't worry about it, it's fine.

At the 45-minute mark, take the lid off and try not to burn the hair off your arms. I have done that a million times and I never seem to learn, but perhaps you will heed my warning. . . .

Put the chicken back in the oven for 20 minutes. You can tell a chicken is cooked by looking at the legs (drumsticks)—if the skin has split away from the joint to the rest of the body, you're in good shape. Throw in the peas in the last ten minutes. Your other veggies will be a little charred and broken down but that's perfect! You can take a fork and pull at the flesh of the leg to make sure it pulls away easily.

Do not take the chicken out of the pot. Take the whole pot out of the oven and let it sit for 10 minutes and then cut it up IN the pot and get all the juices and the veggies mixed up in everything. It should just fall apart. You don't have to do anything fancy with carving this thing, just cut or pull it into pieces, then dish it up with some of that roasted garlic and the juices and veggies and call it dinner.

Save the carcass for soup. I throw the whole thing in a resealable bag and use it later in the week.

# May 22, 2016

I have no idea what to do some days. Change is a giant boulder crashing down a mountain. You have to get out of its way or get flattened, but I keep trying to stand in front of it because I'm so scared of what's about to happen.

Does our memory define who we are? Is that the only measure of a life lived? Or is it something much more delicate and written in the stars—stored on God's "Cloud," as it were. I think it might be. But we depend on remembering what we've done in order to navigate our days. We depend on remembering every small insignificant thing in order to define who we are and what we are. Still, when we lose the ability to know what we've done ten minutes ago, or ten years ago, like Mom has, we ourselves may be able to adjust somehow, but the people around us are hit hard.

For the most part, Mom seems unbothered by what she's lost. She is angry with me, though, because of the people I have hired to help us. She doesn't think I'm being fair or caring in regards to what she wants, which is to be on her own in her house. It just kills me that she's mad at me. I am wound up constantly.

"You just wait," she said as I walked her home last night. "You have no idea how terrible it is to have homeless people in your house." She looks at me in a way that I have never seen her look at me before. Her mouth is pinched in a straight line and her brows knitted together. Her contempt is palpable. It takes my breath away. The women try to stay out of her way, sticking to Dad's old office at night with the baby monitor, but she gets up all night long now, and they need to get up with her.

"They're not homeless, Mom. They're helping us. I don't know what else to do. You can't be alone here anymore. It's not safe for you. I'm doing what you would do for me." This sounds reasonable in my head. Like it would make sense to her. It doesn't.

"I would *never* do this to you. Why in the world aren't I safe? This is ridiculous and I'm moving away. I'm selling everything and moving to a country where I can drive."

"Wouldn't you miss us?"

"Well, I suppose I would, but I can't live like this. This is so awful." She glared at me and let out a long sigh.

"I'm sorry, Mom, but this is the new normal. We just have to be grateful for everything we have. I want you to be able to stay in your own home."

"Are you threatening me?" she said, and stopped in the driveway to face me.

"No, Mom. I just want you to stay home and in order to do that we have to have help. I can't be here with you twenty-four hours a day." I wanted to cry but I didn't.

"So you're going to ship me off if I don't have these bloody ladies in *my* house?" The way she looked at me, it was just not the mother I knew. I tried to breathe through it and not lose my temper. I told her that it was all going to be fine and that we had lots of good things to look forward to. I changed the subject. I talked about Midi and how much stuff we have to get done in the yard. I talked about going to Palm Springs in the fall and or going to England to see Downton Abbey someday.

"That would be nice," she said and we started walking again.

## June 18, 2016

It's been an incredible week here in Maui, writing with Bob Rock. And, yes, that's his real name. He is one of the most naturally gifted musicians I have ever had the

chance to work with in my life, right up there with Ed Cherney and Russ Broom. We've managed to write four pieces of music that may or may not end up on a record, but the process is what always boggles my mind. To create something out of nothing brings so much joy—it's indescribable. It's like a lightning bolt that strikes and makes time itself come to a screeching halt.

The hardest part, of course, is having to be away from Mom. I've spoken to her every day on FaceTime but she always ends up holding the phone up to her ear so I never get to see her! And she sends me texts from her iPad (with a bit of help from Nadine, I'm sure) that are always one very long word.

Hijannmidihadapootodayandwewwntotheriverandbroughtrockshomeforthe gardenloveyouandhopeucomehomeeventually.lovemomm

They always make me so happy. (Well, actually, I feel like bawling when I read them because they're so damn sweet.)

Now I don't even remember what I was talking about . . .

Oh yeah—music and how fantastic it is for the soul. Music saves me every day.

# July 18, 2016

Mom told me the other night that she was going to sue me when "this is all over." Lord, have mercy. She is getting really paranoid and thinks that everyone and their cat is out to get her. The other night she walked over here with my grandmother's old mink coat and told me that "those women were trying to steal it." She wanted me to hide it in the basement.

That same night she came back with a jar of pennies and nickels and dimes and said that she'd split it with me. "There's a few thousand in there that we could use for a trip. . . ."

I could see the companion care worker, Sheri, standing on Mom's front steps and watching where she went, kind enough to give her space and let her walk over here. I'd been sound asleep when she rang the doorbell and I almost went through the ceiling.

It makes me sad.

All of it. The changes and the challenges and the weird things that get put on repeat in her head. She is constantly on the move. She never stops. She folds laundry and walks and putters and moves objects and sits up and looks through the trees for imaginary people. If I didn't have help, I would sink so far down I'd never come up again.

The hardest part, still, is that she is so often mad at me.

She looks at me with such hatred that it takes my breath away. And then it passes, and I see her bubble to the surface of herself again and I wonder how my life got to this place. If you'd told me two years ago that I'd be here, I wouldn't have believed it.

And yet, we fall into so much laughter, feel so much insane gladness and joy. It's such a contrast from one minute to the next and it teaches me constantly. It makes me stronger and humbler and more empathetic and caring and kind. At least I hope it does.

It's just life being life and you've gotta embrace it all with your heart pounding away on your sleeve and a smile on your face . . . and don't forget to cry, because that'll get you through anything.

My mom says tears are God's lubricant to get you through the tight spots. That's a good one.

# August 2, 2016

Grief is a strange thing. It has an actual palpable weight that makes breathing arduous and seems to stifle the heart. At night the weight increases tenfold and pins you to your bed like an unwanted lover.

This whole past year, grief comes and goes like a bratty teenager, oblivious to any kind of caring or responsibility. It moves around in my body silently, like a cancer. I come up for air every few days, to see the sun, to return calls and make meals for my mother, and then I seem to slip back into dull melancholy. It finds cracks in my armour and burns me with the end of its cigarette.

Losing people is what happens to humans. Like a constant drip of an old tap. To try to avoid that loss only leads you to avoid true happiness. We die. But as Snoopy always said, you only die on one day. On the rest of the days you live.

When you don't argue with grief like a drunk husband, much good can come from its stillness. Reflection is so important, time alone, solitude, reckoning. You can't be your best self when you're submerged in useless busy-ness.

Most people choose not to stop long enough to think about how they feel. Most people move from one relationship to the next, one habit to the next, one job to the next, one friend to the next. But in my opinion instant gratification leads you down a lonely path.

Change is taking hold of me and morphing me into a much better version of myself, and that morphing comes with some discomfort. And yes, sometimes it feels like I'm being crushed by that boulder.

Instead of telling that discomfort to go away, I'm going to invite it in. I've learned that it seems to not really like that. It's more used to people who hide from it.

I say let fear and grief sit at your table. Talk to them, give them a cold drink and a sandwich. They simply want to be acknowledged and not ignored. When you ignore them, they just hang around longer.

Mom told me a few months ago that there was an Indian man with a baby in her closet. She said he came and went for a few weeks.

I wanted to say, "Mom, there is no man with a baby in your closet." Instead I asked her what he wanted. She told me he said he wanted to go home.

"What did you say?"

"I told him it was that way . . ."

"And then what?"

"Off he went and he hasn't been back since."

Feel things. Don't be afraid to feel things. That is the whole entire point of all of this.

## September 5, 2016

Fall is my favourite time of year, mainly because it's when we start seriously harvesting the garden. All that waiting for everything to grow is finally over. We dig up potatoes and carrots and beets, and if we're lucky rescue a few bright purple cabbages that the moles always try to eat before we do. Both my parents loved working in the garden and between them they had a wealth of experience. My

maternal and paternal grandparents kept tidy gardens and some of my fondest childhood memories are of wandering along the rows of peas and eating them fresh out of the pods or eating them pods and all. Mom loves working in the garden with me. She loves watching things grow and she loves weeding. Who in their right mind loves weeding? It always amazes me that she can still recognize the difference between the weeds and the vegetables. She can wield that hoe with the precision of a professional gardener. She doesn't shy away from physical labour—in fact, she thrives when she is using a little elbow grease.

Today we dug potatoes for hours, it seemed. I kept having to make Mom stop to take little breaks. I mean, I was exhausted, but she was like the Energizer bunny. I don't think she has any idea how resilient she is. Watching her work in the garden today brought back so many fond memories. She seemed like her old self, the version I still miss, the one who knew all the answers to my questions and solved all the world's mysteries.

We were both pretty pooped by the time we came in, though . . . so I made one of the most comforting and filling of my new "Mom" repertoire.

# ROASTED GARLIC
# AND PARMESAN TOASTED
# BREADCRUMB SPAGHETTI

2 slices whole grain bread (or whatever you have kicking around)

1 box thin pasta—spaghetti, vermicelli, spaghettini—all work

¼ cup extra-virgin olive oil

8–12 garlic cloves (so yes, the whole bulb if you're brave like me and Mom), chopped

salt and pepper

½ tsp chili flakes

1½ cups freshly grated Parmesan cheese (Asiago works too)

a few sprigs of chopped fresh parsley

**It sounds a bit complicated but it's super-fast and super-simple and damn garlicky and good.**

Turn the bread into nice medium-sized crumbs. I find a food processor the easiest way to do it, though a blender works in a pinch.

Boil a pot of water—4 or 5 litres for sure. Salt it very well and add a glug of olive oil. Some people say you shouldn't do this, but I find the oil makes the pasta easy to deal with after you drain the water. While the pasta is cooking (9 or 10 minutes, until al dente), heat the olive oil on medium heat in a large saucepan. (I use a wok.)

Add your chopped garlic. I like to see the chunks, so don't chop it too finely. Once it's in the oil, stir constantly. It will brown very quickly. DO NOT BURN THE GARLIC! Add salt and pepper and chilli flakes, stir stir stir . . . Now throw in the bread crumbs. Stir stir stir . . . After you've stirred it for 4 or 5 minutes, you'll notice it toasting to a beautiful golden brown, which is exactly what you want. Set aside about a half cup of the crumb mixture to sprinkle on top of the pasta right before you serve.

Drain your pasta, reserving ½ cup of the water. Set it aside. Add the pasta directly to your saucepan (or wok) and stir in the garlic mixture. Then add your pasta water a bit at a time to loosen things up slightly and create a bit of a sauce. You don't want it watery, so be mindful to keep it on the thick, pasty side. Add the Parmesan cheese and stir to incorporate it evenly.

When you plate the pasta, add some more cheese, fresh parsley and a bit of the garlic-crumb combo you set aside. I also like to drizzle a little bit of olive oil on top of everything at the end too. Heaven.

## September 12, 2016

After we adopted Lucky the rescue cat I couldn't believe the difference she made in all our lives. I am gobsmacked by how much my mom's focus has shifted from worrying about myriad things to one dear old overweight cat! Lucky sleeps with her every night and they both just *love* it. I'm not really sure who rescued who. . . .

I have read things over the past several years about the importance and value of pets with Alzheimer's patients, but I didn't expect the cat to have such a profound impact on our situation. Lucky seems to know that Mom needs a little extra attention and is more than willing to give it. A noticeable amount of pressure has lifted off my shoulders and I feel better too.

My goal is a simple one: to keep Mom as happy and as safe as humanly possible. She laughs a lot these days and cries much less. She's walking like she's been a Sherpa all her life and eating like a lumberjack, and that is more than I hoped for at this point. I know it will be a lot worse as the weeks and months go by, but for now, Lucky the rescue cat has brought so much love into our home—and a very healthy dose of hope.

## September 28, 2016

People talk about "living in gratitude," but I wonder how many of us are able to truly live our day-to-day lives being thankful for what we have. Like the fact that we are alive and on this magnificent planet, that in this vast universe, we are here, breathing in and out on a tiny speck of wonder, soaring through the cosmos.

I marvel simply looking at my hand. I marvel at tears rolling down my face, at the intricate ability to feel pain and triumph. I marvel at the concept of love, its infinite power, its endless good.

WOW. (Mom pointed out the other day that WOW was MOM upside down.)

Living in gratitude is about HOW we see things. Your intentions hold incredible power. Be mindful of them. Point them in a good direction. Be earnest. Be the kind of person you want to attract into your own life. Humility takes incredible strength.

And although this life is filled with enormous grief and sadness and challenges and depression and loss and death, it is also filled with promise. We easily lose sight of that when things go sideways, and they often do. Life is going to be hard a lot of the time and that's okay. You can do it.

Living in gratitude involves a lot more than saying you're grateful. It is a way of existing. In poker you often hear the phrase "all in." Living in a real state of gratitude means just that: every second has to be *all in*. Being grateful for pain lessens the hurt. Being grateful for loss may not make any sense, but it's a way of allowing your heart and mind to let things go instead of dragging them with you.

It's interesting to me how much I gain from letting things go, how much I learn that is directly linked to how often I fail. Every single time you don't get it right is like a building block to becoming a better version of yourself.

Flying is falling.

We spend so much time worrying about dying, and that causes us to worry about living. So let the universe have its way with you.

You are a piece of it all. Infinite. Boundless. Indivisible.

# October 5, 2016

I had a really difficult evening with my mom. Every week it seems we enter a new phase of this incredibly cruel disease.

More and more frequently, she brings up the issue of people stealing from her. It's almost always about money. Ten days ago, she wandered over to my house at close to midnight, rang the doorbell and, when I answered, handed me a plastic bag filled with rolled-up toonies. (My dad must have had them stashed in their closet.) She told me the homeless ladies were trying to steal them and asked me to hide them, which I did.

A few days later, she told me they were gone, that someone had taken them. I reminded her that she had brought them to me to keep.

"Oh yeah. I seem to recall that."

"We'll take them to the bank so they're safe." I thought that would make her feel better, but nope.

"The banks aren't safe."

"They're safer than my house."

"Why do you have my money?"

"You brought it here for safekeeping."

Living in gratitude is about HOW we see things.

I won't bore you with the remaining thirty minutes of the conversation.

Last night she told me—again—that she didn't want any ladies in the house anymore. That she used to like them but not since they've been stealing from her.

The *coins* again. (I need to add that her fortune in toonies amounted to about $200.) She is fixated on them. She goes over and over it in her mind, how all the money she has to her name has been stolen from her.

Alzheimer's pounds all sense into nonsense.

I reminded her that she'd brought them to me a few weeks earlier and that we were going to take them to the bank at some point.

"Are you saying that I am crazy, Jann? How stupid do you think I am?"

The blood rushes to my face and my heart picks up speed. My feelings are hurt. I know they shouldn't be, but I can't separate my idea of Mom from this version.

"I'm not saying that for a second!" My voice rises and I start to swallow a lot.

Mom becomes frantic. "Why in the world do you hate me SO much?"

I am trying to stay calm but I'm getting angry because I'm helpless, and I know she will forget this whole conversation in five minutes. "I don't hate you at all! I would never, ever, hate you, Mom. You just forgot you gave me the coins. I would never steal them from you."

She sets the dinner I've just made her aside and says she's going home. "I don't have to put up with this!"

"Mom, please sit back down and eat your dinner."

"I'm moving to Vancouver."

"Won't you miss me and Midi?"

"Yes. Yes, I will." Her brain clicks into another gear. "Is this chicken?"

"Yes, it's chicken and the potatoes are from our garden."

"Did we plant a garden?"

"You planted it with me. We had a good day."

"We did have a good day. It was a nice day for it, wasn't it?" She cuts a piece of chicken off the bone and gives it to Belle, our big dog. She pretends that I don't see her do it.

"That's for you, not the dog, Mom."

"It won't kill her to have a piece of chicken."

"You're right, it won't."

"I can't have those ladies at my house anymore. They'll have to find another place to live."

"Okay." What else can I say? My heart is still pounding.

I miss my mom, desperately at times, but even so I'm glad to have this version of her still here with me. I'm trying to learn how to find a language between us that doesn't infuriate me and hurt her feelings. It's like a dance. A dance with music that changes its beat every few seconds.

Mom stops talking now as she often does. She's silent a lot of the time—unless her brain puts her on that crazy-ass spinning wheel. I give her a big bowl of Jell-O and she asks me if I made it from scratch and I tell her, no, that it came from a box.

Then she asks me if it's 1915. I tell her it is.

"See," she says. "I'm not that crazy. . . ."

## October 28, 2016

I am a mother to my mother. It's a massive learning curve, not only because I didn't have children of my own, but because there isn't a handbook telling me what I should or shouldn't be doing. Alzheimer's is a different disease for every single person it inhabits. Everything is a trial by fire.

My biggest enemy is patience, or rather, the lack thereof. I feel myself crumble as my mom's memory crumbles. I feel part of myself die a little bit more every time she forgets something new. It's as if we are still joined by the cord that connected us all those lifetimes ago.

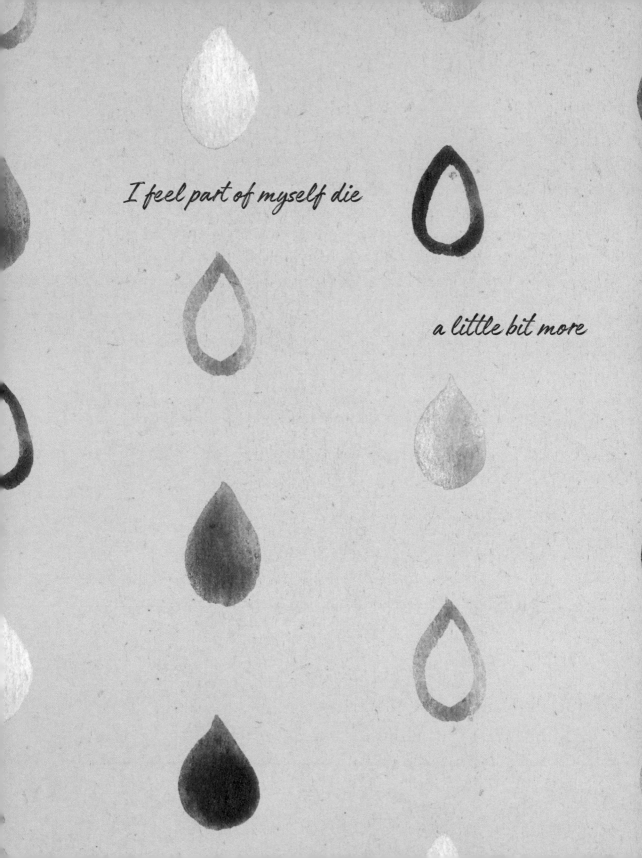

I feel part of myself die

a little bit more

every time she forgets

something new.

Last night when she was here for dinner, she got up and said she had to use the washroom. She made her way over to the door to the deck and was trying to go outside. I asked her where she was going and she said, "I'm trying to get to the bathroom."

"The bathroom is this way."

"It is?"

"Don't you remember the little side bathroom?" I got up and walked her back toward the bathroom door and she acted like she had never ever set foot in that part of my house before.

"Well, this is a cute room," she said, looking around. She had her arms folded across her chest.

How, from one day to the next, can things simply disappear?

"Have you always had this?" she said to me with an eyebrow raised.

"Yes."

"Have I used this bathroom?"

"Yes."

So I am a mother to my mother, and I don't know what I'm doing half the time. I don't know if I'm doing the right thing or the wrong thing, making things better or making things worse.

I lost my temper a few hours ago. Mom decided to take the leather straps off the dog bag I carry Midi in. I don't why she thought she needed to do that, and she doesn't know why either. But I can't use the bag without the straps and, more aggravating still, I had just had them replaced. I huffed and puffed and stormed out of her house and across the driveway to my house with Midi under my arm in the bag with no straps. I was being impulsive and bratty and stupid and I knew I was before "WHY DID YOU TAKE THE STRAPS OFF?!" even came out of my mouth. I saw her head drop and I wanted to stab myself in the eyeball. I'd hurt her feelings and for what?

Donna, another of our care workers, told me that she would look for them. "Don't worry," she said. "We'll find them."

And they found them two minutes after I'd stomped out the door, sitting on the kitchen counter.

I told Mom how sorry I was a dozen times. "Would a thousand dollars make up for it?"

And she kidded right back, without missing a beat, "How about five thousand?"

# November 26, 2016

I don't know my mom very well anymore. I hate even writing down these words. I hurl myself back in time to find scraps of who she used to be wandering around in my early memories.

Emily Dickinson wrote a poem well over a hundred years ago and its haunting opening verse reads:

Pain has an element of blank;
It cannot recollect

When it began, or if there were
A day when it was not.

I can't remember the day when my mother starting becoming someone new, someone changed and altered. I can't remember that precious moment when I started saying the longest goodbye of my life. I wrote a song about it a few months ago with Bob Rock and I'm still having a hard time listening to the demo.

When I was away these past two weeks, I felt riddled with guilt and I felt so relieved at the same time. It's nearly impossible to have these two very different emotions mingling inside my heart. They fight with each other like a married couple on their third bottle of wine. Emily goes on to say:

It has no future but itself,
Its infinite realms contain
Its past, enlightened to perceive
New periods of pain.

*New periods of pain* indeed. I watched Mom as she napped on my couch last night. I needed to feed us something but I was tired out from travelling. There wasn't a lot of choices. I still have yet to grab a few groceries (maybe tomorrow).

I ended up throwing some spaghetti in a pot of boiling water and dumping on some canned tomato sauce for us to have for dinner—not one of my better creations.

The TV was on in the background and Midi was snoring. It was just one of those moments that I locked onto.

I stood there in front of my sleeping mom holding our crappy supper on a tray and I was torn between letting her rest and feeding her. I wished that I could have stayed in that ONE spot forever. I wished I could have stayed in the quiet and the calm, where this *thing* wasn't going to get worse and that my mom didn't have to endure the indignity of forgetting who she was.

When my dad was still alive, I remember Mom calling me for the millionth time to come over and fix the remote control for the television. I rolled my eyes and told her that I would come over as soon as I could. (I live one hundred feet away, so not a big deal.) When I got there, they both looked at me like I was going to beat them up, and that made me feel terrible. They had heard the anger in my voice and they felt bad that I'd had to interrupt my writing to come and help them. (I'm an asshole.) Anyhow, they handed me an old remote for a TV they didn't even HAVE anymore. I found the right one in the bag of dog food.

You gotta laugh.

Mom said to me, "Jann, you're the only one freaking out. We would have found the g.d. thing eventually."

Very true. I was and am the only one freaking out. My mom is mostly calm and funny and loving life. She doesn't know what she has and I'm grateful for that.

Finally, I woke her up and said, "Dinner is served!"

"That looks wonderful," she said smiling.

I'm trying to focus on what I have, and not what I don't have.

# December 15, 2016

When we weighed Mom a few months ago, she was only 104 pounds, and her doctor basically said that I needed to get her to eat, and it didn't matter what—she *i needed to get her to eat...*

needed to eat everything. I wish I had a doctor telling me that: "Jann, we need you to eat whatever you want, whenever you want. It's for your own good!" I don't think I'll live to hear those words. It's been challenging, to say the least, to put some pounds on my mother while trying to drop some pounds myself.

A lot of people send me articles about things that might be helpful to me and Mom, especially in the dietary department. I've lost track of how often I'm sent some info on the magical benefits of coconut oil, for instance. But what the heck, I started using coconut oil on everything, eating the stuff by the boatload. It tastes great, it is the good kind of fat and it has a very high "burn" threshold, which makes it great for quickly searing things like fish or onions, or making stir-fries. As far as what it does for memory? That's up in the air. People swear on a stack of Bibles that it makes a big difference in their loved ones who are suffering from dementia and Alzheimer's, so I use it just in case what they say is true. I know that doesn't sound very rational or scientific, but it's not doing any harm, and it might do some good. Mom says to me at least once a week that she thinks the coconut oil is working. It kind of makes my heart ache.

Mom has gained five pounds in the last couple of months. And I'm slowly losing weight: I figured doing something positive about taking care of myself might help me tackle my depression, which comes and goes like a bad relationship. I've been working out hard and eating REAL food, which is exactly what I feed Mom. REAL FOOD. I make sure she has lots of good carbs and I take it very easy on the rice and potatoes and the bread. Otherwise we eat the same things. Eating good food is changing both of us. I have to be at my very best to keep up with this woman.

Here are a couple of the recipes that helped me bulk her up.

# CHEDDAR, ONION AND
# MUSHROOM QUICHE

2 tbsp butter

½ cup diced white onion

1 cup sliced mushrooms

salt and pepper

5 eggs

¼ cup half-and-half or
whipping cream.
(Don't use milk here as
it makes the quiche too
watery.)

1 green onion, chopped

1 cup shredded cheddar
cheese, or cheese of
your choice—they will
ALL work fine

1 frozen pie crust

Preheat your oven to 350°F.

Set a frying pan over medium heat. Add the butter. Add the onions
and mushrooms and salt and pepper to taste, and cook until soft.

In a large mixing bowl, beat all 5 eggs and cream with a fork until
thoroughly combined. Add the cooked onions and mushrooms, green
onion and half the cheese to the eggs and fold in well.

Lay the crust in the pie plate and poke it with a fork to keep it from
puffing. Pour in the egg mixture and sprinkle the remaining cheese on
top. Bake on the middle rack of the oven for 35 minutes.

# EASY FOUR-CHEESE MAC

2 cups dry macaroni
pasta

2 tbsp butter

2 tbsp flour

1 ½ cups milk

salt and pepper

½ tsp cayenne

½ cup panko crumbs

1 cup shredded old
cheddar

½ cup crumbled blue
cheese

½ cup grated Parmesan
cheese

½ cup grated Swiss
cheese

Preheat the oven to 375°F. Cook your pasta, drain and set aside.

In a saucepan, melt butter over medium heat. Add flour to make a paste, stirring constantly to keep it from burning. Whisk in your milk and bring it to a simmer, stirring until it bubbles and thickens. Add all your cheeses, salt and pepper and cayenne and make sure everything is melted and stirred together.

Put your cooked pasta into a casserole dish, pour the cheese sauce over the pasta and stir together. Sprinkle the panko crumbs evenly over the top. Bake for 15 minutes, let cool for 15 minutes and serve.

# December 24, 2016

Mom and I are sitting here waiting for everybody to arrive. She is surprised that we are having Christmas *again*. We *just* had it.

We have a few hours to ourselves to drink tea and eat goodies, and she is mowing through the shortbread and caramels and chocolate like there is no tomorrow. We have *A Madea Christmas* playing in the background and every now and then Mom asks me if Madea is a man. Makes me laugh every damn time.

She also keeps asking me if there is anything else she can do. Alzheimer's folks are very task-oriented, or my mom is, anyway. She always wants to be busy and doing things. She wants to be purposeful. Don't we all . . .

Just now she decided she needs to bring in some firewood. She grabs a couple of logs at a time and goes in and out the patio door. It's quite something watching her can-do spirit. She simply does not stop. So far she has folded clothes, mopped the floor and shovelled the driveway. I feel slightly guilty. No, seriously—I do. It's like having my own personal Molly Maid. I didn't even need the floors mopped, but she was so determined to be useful I couldn't say no.

I totally understand it. I am terrible at sitting and doing nothing. I don't like lying on a beach for more than twenty minutes, for instance, and I'm pretty sure I get it from her.

She finally sits down again and I'm going to try and keep her in one spot for the next hour. It's stopped snowing but while it was coming down it was simply beautiful. She's already mentioned needing to go out and shovel again. You gotta laugh. Maybe it's time to start pouring the eggnog and rum!

I'm so grateful for all the lessons this past year. I'm grateful for the mishaps and the mistakes. I'm grateful for the failures and the heartbreaks and the obstacles.

There is so much joy. There is so much hope.

I truly believe there are a lot of things to look forward to in 2017.

Keep your wits about you.

Be spontaneous.

Be easy on yourself.

Rejoice!

Rejoice!

MERRY CHRISTMAS, HAPPY HANUKAH!

Whatever your beliefs be, I hope goodness is at the heart of them all.

## January 1 at 2:18pm

Hello, 2017.

What are you going to do with me?

I find myself at an interesting crossroads in my life. Well, more of a raging, multi-lane intersection. The last two years have been like watching a slow-motion car crash knowing there isn't a bloody thing I can do to stop it.

We all have times that seem to explode with "happenings"—a succession of years that pound and punch and mete out the unexpected and leave one feeling

quite helpless indeed. And then comes the calm, the reflection, the time for the decision making that one has to do in order to turn the chaos into some sort of manageable order.

It's all daunting, but doable.

For the first time in twenty-five years or so, I am alone in this house. No one to answer to, or argue with, or sort out or save or hoist or drag down the road behind me. It's weird and wonderful and probably the best thing that's ever happened to me. I can breathe. I didn't even know I wasn't breathing—that's the really funny thing.

Life can become a complete blur without you even knowing it.

WE. DON'T. STOP.

My father's death was sad, but not unexpected. It was slow and tedious and terrifying. But people die. It was an amazing experience and I learned a lot about myself and the people around me.

My mother keeps spiralling into the abyss of Alzheimer's but, thankfully, she is the only one who doesn't know. Alzheimer's is a disease that hits the people who have to watch it happen much harder at first than the people who are losing themselves. You have to laugh loud and long or you won't survive it, *and* you have to lean on your friends. You have to ask for help. You can't do it alone.

And you have to stay in the moment you're in and not live even one single hour in the future. NOW. NOW. NOW.

That is Alzheimer's.

Hmmn, what else?

I'm finishing a novel, starting a new album, developing a TV series, planning tours, fixing my body, being kind to myself and putting myself out there in the universe by embracing whatever it is that awaits my participation. I'm baking and painting and walking and exercising and doing yoga and praying and thinking. And most of all, appreciating my dear-heart friends and the brilliant creative people I work with day in and day out.

But I try not to do everything at the same time.

Also, music is everything. It has revealed my own soul to me.

## February 1, 2017

Alzheimer's doesn't take big things away, at least not at first. It takes very small things that don't seem all that important until you string them together. It's a disease that seems to cut the dog's tail off one inch at a time, which is just cruel and malicious if you ask me. Mom doesn't know how to make coffee anymore, or use a phone, or turn on the TV. She has no idea how long she was married, or how many kids she has or if she still has a mother or how to turn the knobs in the shower. It's all just lost. She doesn't really know how to use her blow dryer or open a can or turn on the gas stove. Alzheimer's takes away very small things.

Every single day, some part of her brain walks off into the sunset and waves goodbye. She doesn't know that she's unwell. She doesn't know that there is a dark shadow creeping through her skull wiping away important information. Her mind tells her over and over again that she is perfectly fine.

That is a blessing, for sure. The bliss that comes with her deep forgetfulness makes me truly grateful. She still knows who everybody is, she knows how to laugh and she knows how to walk down the road and eat a Dairy Queen sundae. She watches

the news with me at night and always remarks that things will get better. She told me that life was upside down in the thirties, too, and that all the countries got together and fought to put things right again. That made me feel hopeful.

"Life goes on," she says to me as she colours in her book. She's presently working on a little dog walking on a rainbow. Very fitting . . .

She needs my help to put the cap back on the markers. That breaks my heart a bit.

I told Mom I was worried about the world and she told me to just live my life and help other people—that that was what it was all about. "If everybody helped everybody, the world would be perfect." Sage advice from a person who has been through a lot—a few wars, a few depressions, poverty, abuse, loss of every description. And yet, she is of good cheer. "You have to keep going no matter what," she tells me as she looks out the window at two squirrels racing up a tree. "He should spend a few hours every day watching squirrels—that would help him."

I think she's talking about Trump and that makes me kind of snort.

"You never know, Mom. That might help him."

And then she says, "Well, they must have squirrels on the planet he comes from."

She hands another marker to me so I can take the cap off.

*Final words. Well, nothing is ever final, but here goes.*

I don't know what the future holds for me or my mom. I have a few ideas as to what's going to unfold but they aren't worth spreading out on the table and staring at for months on end. There are far too many uncertainties and far too many things that will remain completely unknown until the very last second.

That's what life is good at—being mysterious and unpredictable.

My mom doesn't know what she did or said two minutes ago. Things are lost almost as soon as they are experienced. I've learned to let all her fleeting memories float up into the air. I tried too long to be her memory and her intentions and her sense of reason and all I managed to do was exhaust my patience and make myself anxious. It has made me very depressed at times to watch her personality and her abilities diminish. It's like starting from square one every morning. Remember *Groundhog Day*? I now live in that movie. But I've learned to embrace who she is, and not hang on to who she was. That's one thing I have really learned, because anything else is too painful and frustrating.

As my mother's daughter and caregiver, I have to stay in the moment that my mom lives in. I have to hold her hand and go down the road that she is on without question or hesitation. I've learned that it's liberating to surrender. Surrendering is not giving up, not at all. Surrendering to Alzheimer's means giving up that damaging emotional battle to be right. Marianne Williamson, the wonderful spiritual guru and author, wrote: "Ego says, 'Once everything falls into place, I'll feel peace.' Spirit says, 'Find your peace and then everything will fall into place.'" I'll never forget reading those sentences and how they resonated with every part of my life. I don't want to spend my life forcing everything into the right place anymore.

When this all started, I thought that if I rolled up my sleeves and went to war with Alzheimer's, I could buy my mom some time and keep that dreaded disease at bay. That's not the way it works. The harder I pushed, the harder my mother pulled. I found out rather quickly how determined she and her Alzheimer's were going to be.

I had to adapt to meet my mother's disease head on, and that change has affected my entire life. It's changed the way I approach my work and how I interact with my friends and even how I have treated my body these past few years. I feel like I am as changed as my mother is. We have somehow managed to morph ourselves into some kind of superhero in order to cope with our day-to-day lives. I couldn't remain the person I was. I had to alter pretty much everything about my life. It's been scary and sad, but it's also been exhilarating.

I know that things are going to get worse for my mom—that she will succumb to this thing eventually—but I still feel a wonderful sense of hopefulness. I don't know a lot, but I know that we are going to be some version of fine. That I am going to be fine and that Mom will be cushioned by a whole lot of love from a whole lot of people. It's an amazing thing to know that so many human beings are cheering for us, and sharing their strength and understanding. To know that we aren't alone on this road has meant the world to me. When we go on our morning walks down the road, I tell Mom about all the people who think she is so cool and so funny and so beautiful. Her face lights up and for a brief moment she looks so familiar to me. I cherish those few minutes more than I can express. Mom rises up out of her Alzheimer's and does her best to show me that she's in there, and that she is intact. I can see it in the curve of her mouth and the setting of her perfect jawline, so strong and capable. Those moments help to keep my fears away, they really do. Somehow, Mom has managed to show me that she is winning despite how things may outwardly appear. It is truly a gift to have those tiny bits of a reprieve to ease my worries.

As we go forward, those moments when she reveals herself will become fewer and farther between, but that doesn't mean I am going to lose faith.

My dad always used to say, "If you're failing you're trying." I think about that a lot these days and reflect on what it has meant at different times in my life. And I keep reminding myself that what's going on with me and my mom is just life. It's the obstacles that teach us to be better versions of ourselves. It's the hardships and the sadness that show us the beauty of joy and happiness. You can't have one without the other.

So Alzheimer's and I have decided that we have to work together in order to be as well as we can be and live our best lives.

No matter what happens, I'm going to be feeding my mother.

[ACKNOWLEDGEMENTS]

*Thank You*

I am so grateful to the amazing group of caregivers who look after Mom with me seven days a week, pretty much twenty-four hours a day. We rely on, and cannot live without, your humour, grace and patience, your kindness and generosity of spirit. Without you, my brothers, Pat and Duray, and I couldn't manage. A heartfelt thank you to Ginny Smale, Donna Marie Dillman, Donna Godlonton, Montana Hancocks, Sheila Silla and Jenna Cameron.

I also want to thank Theresa deWaal, Laurel Frezell, Bev Oldham, Lisa Almond, Pat Hillcof and Sherry Lewis, my wonderful women friends who have helped me out whenever something came up over the last few years—when I had to travel unexpectedly or was in some other kind of a bind. These fine souls showed up with food in hand and smiles on their faces! Speaking of food, thanks to my old friend and cooking pro Julie Van Rosendaal for making sure that somebody else besides me could follow my recipes.

And, lastly, I would be completely lost without my friend and fearless leader, Nadine (Deneen, as Mom calls her) Beauchesne. She manages to keep us keeping on with determination and impeccable organizational skills. Nadine, you always go above and beyond to make sure Mom is having loads of fun and that she is safe and well.

# [RECIPES]